A National Agenda for Geriatric Education

A National Agenda for Geriatric Education

White Papers

Susan M. Klein, DNSc, RN
Editor

Springer Publishing Company

Disclaimer

The Bureau of Health Professions of the Health Resources and Services Administration has a mission to provide leadership to improve the training, distribution, utilization, and quality of personnel required to staff the nation's health care system. The following White Papers were prepared for the invitaional National Forum on Geriatric Education and Training, held in 1995. The opinions expressed herein are the views of the authors and do not necessarily reflect the official position of the Health Resources and Services Administration. The U.S. Government does not endorse or favor any specific commercial product. Trade or proprietary names appearing in this publication are used only because they are considered essential in the context of the reports herein.

Published in 1997

97 98 99 00 01 / 5 4 3 2 1

Library of Congress Cataloging-in-Publication Data

A national agenda for geriatric education: white papers / [edited by] Susan M. Klein.
p. cm.
Includes bibliographical references.
ISBN 0-8261-9970-4 (alk. paper)
1. Geriatrics—Study and teaching—United States. I. Klein, Susan M.
[DNLM: 1. Geriatrics—education—United States. 2. Geriatric Nursing—education—United States. WT 18 N2767 1997]
RC952.5.N37 1997
618.97'0071'173—dc21
DNLM/DLC
for Library of Congress 97-4390
CIP

Printed in the United States of America

Contents

3

SOCIAL WORK

Barbara Berkman, DSW, LICSW, Rose Dobrof, DSW,
Lois Harry, PhD, and Joan Damron-Rodriguez, PhD

4

LONG-TERM CARE

Margaret Dimond, PhD, RN, FAAN, Donna Lind Infeld, PhD,
Alice Kethley, PhD, and Eric Pfeiffer, MD

Contributors

PROJECT DIRECTOR
Bernice A. Parlak, MSW Chief
Interdisciplinary, Geriatrics and Allied
Health Branch
Bureau of Health Professions
Health Resources & Services Administration

EDITOR/PROJECT CO-DIRECTOR
Susan M. Klein, HM, DNSc, RN
Public Health Analyst
Interdisciplinary, Geriatrics and Allied
Health Branch
Bureau of Health Professions
Health Resources & Services Administration

Lynne Anker-Unnever, MPA
St. Joseph
Health Care System
New Mexico
Managed Care

Barbara Berkman, DSW, LICSW
Massachusetts General Hospital
Harvard GEC
Social Work

Marie Bernard, MD
Veterans Administration Medical Center
Oklahoma City
University of Oklahoma
Oklahoma GEC
Interdisciplinary Education

Kathleen Buckwalter, PhD, RN, FAAN
The University of Iowa
Nursing

Ann H. Cary, PhD, MPH, RN, A-CCC
George Mason University
Public Health

Richard Connelly, PhD
Veterans Administration Medical Center
Salt Lake City
University of Utah
Intermountain West GEC
Interdisciplinary Education

Joan Damron-Rodriguez, Ph.D.
Veterans Administration Medical Center
West Los Angeles
University of California, Los Angeles
California GEC
Social Work

Margaret Dimond, PhD, RN, FAAN
University of Washington
Long Term Care

Rose Dobrof, DSW
Hunter College, City University of New York
Hunter/Mt. Sinai GEC
Social Work

Pricilla Ebersole, PhD, RN, FAAN
San Francisco State University
Nursing

Terry Fulmer, PhD, RN, C, FAAN
Columbia University
New York GEC
Nursing

Jennie Chin Hansen, MSN, RN
On-Lok, Inc.
Stanford GEC
Managed Care

Lois Harry, PhD
University of Nevada, Reno
Nevada GEC
Social Work

Neil Henderson, PhD
University of South Florida
Ethnogeriatrics

Donna Lind Infeld, PhD
George Washington University
Long Term Care

Alice Kethley, PhD
Benjamin Rose Institute
Long Term Care

Linda Kuder, PhD
University of Kentucky
Ohio Valley Appalachia Regional GEC
Interdisciplinary Education

Ronald Lankford, MD
Private Consultant
Kentucky
Managed Care

Melvina McCabe, MD
University of New Mexico
New Mexico GEC
Ethnogeriatric

Joan B. McDowell, PhD, CRNP, FAAN
University of Pittsburgh
GEC of Pennsylvania
Nursing

Joanna Mellor, DSW
Hunter/MT. Sinai GEC
Interdisciplinary Education

F. Ellen Netting, PhD, ACSW
Virginia Commonwealth University
Case Management

Linda Norman, MSN, RN
Vanderbilt University
Interdisciplinary Education

Edwin J. Olsen, MD, MBA
Veterans Administration Medical Center Miami
University of Miami
Miami Are GEC
Managed Care

Janet Olszewski, MSW
Michigan Department of Public Health
Managed Care

James T. Pacala, MD, MS
University of Minnesota
Minnesota GEC
Case Management

Richard Della Penna, MD
Kaiser Permanente Medical Group
San Diego, California
Managed Care

Eric Pfeiffer, MD
University of South Florida
Long Term Care

Thomas Prohaska, PhD
University of Illinois at Chicago
Illinois GEC Network
Public Health

Joan Quinn, MS, RN, FAAN
Blue Cross and Blue Shield of Connecticut
Case Management

Linda Redford, PhD RN,
University of Kansas
Case Management

Joanne Schwartzberg, MD
American Medical Association
Case Management

Veronica J. Scott, MD, MPH
Meharry Medical College
Meharry Consortium GEC
Ethnogeriatrics

Leopold G. Selker, PhD
Evanston Hospital Corporation
Illinois
Allied & Associated Health

Myrna Silverman, PhD
University of Pittsburgh
GEC of Pennsylvania
Public Health

Melissa Talamantes, MS
University of Texas at San Antonio
Ethnogeriatrics

Ruth Ann Tsukuda, MPH, BSN, RN
Portland Veterans Administration
Medical Center
Oregon GEC
Interdisciplinary Education

Steven P. Wallace, PhD
University of California, Los Angeles
California GEC
Public Health

Ann L. Wall, PhD, RN, FAAN
University of Michigan
Nursing

Monika White, PhD
Senior Health and Peer Counseling
Case Management

C. Edwin Webb, PharmD, MPH
American Association of
Colleges of Pharmacy

May L. Wykle, PhD, RN, FAAN
Case Western Reserve University
Western Reserve GEC
Nursing

Barbara Yee, PhD
University of Texas Medical Branch at Galveston
Texas Consortium GEC
Ethnogeriatrics

Gwen Yeo, PhD
Stanford University
Stanford GEC
Ethnogeriatrics

REVIEWERS

Amanda Barusch, DSW
University of Utah
Social Work

Mathy D. Mezey, PhD, RN, FAAN
New York University
Columbia University - New York GEC
Long Term Care

Renee Solomon, DSW
Columbia University
Social Work

Foreword

Current age graphing of the U.S. population follows the rise of the large bubble of baby boomers toward old age. The aging of this generation in particular is precipitating a review by many societal institutions of the country's readiness to meet the late-life needs of this population. The preparedness of the nation's health professions to provide geriatric primary and long-term care in an effective and efficient manner within a rapidly changing health care environment is also under scrutiny.

The need for adequately trained health care providers is urgent. At present no health care profession meets the minimum number of geriatrically trained personnel necessary to adequately meet the unique health care needs of the elderly. The numbers of persons with functional limitations, Alzheimer's Disease or other dementing illness is increasing, and health professionals must be prepared to find new and better ways to prevent or treat these and many other conditions that steal personal independence and rob approximately one of every five older Americans of productive, satisfying lives.

What directions should schools of the health professions take regarding geriatric education as 56 million baby boomers face advancing age and the elderly population becomes significantly more ethnically and racially diverse? In a time of diminishing resources, are the schools of the health professions able to respond adequately to the demand for competent care of older adults? Responses to these and other focal questions are being generated through the Geriatric Education Futures Project. This innovative, open-ended, multiphase project, initiated in 1994 by the Bureau of Health Professions, Health Resources and Services Administration, is designed as an organic system, building synergy from phase to phase. The goal of the project is to promote and improve geriatric education in the health professions and thereby respond to a national health care need.

Phase One of the project produced the publication *A National Agenda for Geriatric Education, Volume I: White Papers*. The 11 papers were developed by Study Groups of recognized leaders in their fields. They provide a base of fact, vision, and policy recommendations for the continuous improvement of geriatric education. Phase Two of the invitational National Forum on Geriatric Education and Training was convened to explore the parameters that define the needs in geriatric education; assess the outcomes of programmatic approaches to date; examine funding strategies; and identify the factors that limit or enhance the education and training of health care professionals in geriatrics and gerontology. The Forum brought together experts in geriatric education, funding agents, providers, consumers, educators in the health professions, and policymakers. They also affirmed the work of the Study Groups. Phase Two produced the publication, *A National Agenda for Geriatric Education, Volume 2: Forum Report* available from the U.S. Department of Health and Human Services.

The work of Phase Three is currently under way and comprises three major initiatives: the development of a formal Agenda for Action: Strategic Recommendation for Geriatric Education replete with a promotions package to be disseminated widely throughout the field; development of interprofessional collaboratives to prompt joint ventures between organizations to meet common education and training goals; and the publication of journal articles, texts, and other related materials including an annual Tracer Reports to track the achievements of the collaboratives and accomplishment of the White Paper recommendations. A second National Forum for Geriatric Education and Training is planned for the year 2000.

Key to the ongoing success of the Geriatric Education Futures Project is the foundation laid in the work of the Study Group members. Appreciation is extended to these highly skilled and deeply dedicated professionals whose collaborative work produced papers that are both pragmatic and visionary. The breadth of knowledge, experience, and wisdom ensconced in the whole of the Study Groups makes the 11 *White Papers* produced in Phase One critically important to further strategic planning. Their clear vision continues to provide structure and guidance for a variety of health care educators, policymakers, federal agencies, foundations, and accreditation bodies in the implementation of a collaborative agenda for action in support of geriatric education and better health for older Americans.

BERNICE A. PARLAK
Acting Director
Division of Associated, Dental,
and Public Health Professions

Director
Geriatric Education Futures Project

Acronyms

AADS American Association of Dental Schools
AAGP American Association for Geriatric Psychiatry
AAMC Association of American Medical Colleges
AARP American Association for Retired People
ABFP American Board of Family Practice
ABIM American Board of Internal Medicine
ABMS American Board of Medical Specialists
ACGME Accreditation Council for Graduate Medical Education
ACGOM Accreditation Council for Graduate Osteopathic Medicine
ADGAP Association of Directors of Geriatric Academic Programs
ADA American Dental Association
ADHA American Dental Hygiene Association
AEGD Advanced Education on General Dentistry
AFAR American Federation for Aging Research
AGD Academy of General Dentistry
AGF Academic Geriatrician Faculty
AGS American Geriatric Society
AHCPR Agency for Health Care Policy and Research
AHECs Area Health Education Centers
AMA American Medical Association
AMDA American Medical Director Association
ANA American Nurses Association
AoA Administration on Aging
AOA American Osteopathic Association
APA American Psychological Association
ASA American Society on Aging
ASAHP American Society of Allied Health Profession
ASGD American Society for Geriatric Dentistry
AUPHA Association of University Programs in Health Administration
BHPr Bureau of Health Professions
BLS Bureau of Laboratory Statistics
BSW Bachelors in Social Work
CAAHEP Commission on Accreditation of Allied Health Education Programs
CAQGM Certification of Added Qualifications in Geriatric Medicine
CBLTC Community Based Long Term Care
CD-ROM Computer disk-Read only memory
CE Continuing Education
CGA Comprehensive Geriatric Assessment
CME Continuing Medical Education
CMHS Center for Mental Health Services
COGME Council On Graduate Medical Education

CQI Continuous Quality Improvement
CSWE Council of Social Work Education
DHHS Department of Health and Human Services
DRGs Diagnostic Related Groups
DVA Department of Veteran Affairs
EFDAs Expanded Function Dental Assistants
FTPs Faculty Training Projects
GCNs Geriatric Care Networks
GCNS Geriatric Clinical Nurse Specialists
GECs Geriatric Education Centers
GHAA Group Health Association of America
GME Graduate Medical Education
GNP Geriatric Nurse Practitioners
GPR General Practice Residency
GRECC Geriatric Research Education and Clinical Center
HCFA Health Care Financing Administration
HMOs Health Maintenance Organizations
HRSA Health Resources and Services Administration
IOM Institute of Medicine
ITTG Interdisciplinary Team Training in Geriatrics
ITTP Interdisciplinary Team Training Program
JAMA Journal of the American Medical Association
JCAHC Joint Commission for Accreditation of Healthcare Organizations
LCME Liaison Committee on Medical Education
LTC Long Term Care
MDS Minimum Data Set
MFP Minority Fellowship Program
MSW Master in Social Work
NAAAA National Association of Area Agencies on Aging
NASW National Association of Social Work
NCCC National Chronic Care Consortium
NIA National Institute on Aging
NIDR National Institute of Dental Research
NIDRR National Institute on Disabilities, Rehabilitation and Research
NIH National Institute of Health
NIMH National Institute of Mental Health
NLM National Library of Medicine
NSIMMP National Study of Internal Medicine Manpower
NSOH National Survey of Oral Healthy
OBRA Omnibus Budget Reconciliation Act
PPOs Preferred Provider Organizations
PPRC Physician Payment Review Commission
PTA Physical Therapist Assistant
PT Physical Therapy
QA Quality Assurance
QI Quality Improvement
RBRVS Resource Board Relative Value System
RFAs Request for Applications
RRC Residency Review Committee
RWJF Robert Wood Johnson Foundation
SHMOs Social Health Maintenance Organizations
SWFDP Social Work Faculty Development Program
TBCUs Traditionally Black Colleges and Universities
TEFRA Tax Equity and Fiscal Responsibility Act
TNH Teaching Nursing Home
TQM Total Quality Management
USMLE US Medical Licenses Examiner
VA Veterans Administration
WHNPs Women's Health Nurse Practitioners

Introduction

An Aging Nation

Currently over 12% of the U.S. population is 65 years of age or older, and by the year 2030 they will comprise 21% of the population. Most of the projected increase in the 65 plus population is due to the aging of 76 million baby boomers born between 1946 and 1964. During 2010–2030, the number of older adults will grow by an average of 2.8 percent annually. The elderly population is also becoming more ethnically and racially diverse. Between the years 1994–2030, races other than White will increase in proportion from 10% to 20% of the elderly. Similarly, Hispanic elderly are expected to grow in proportion to other older adults from 4% to 16%.

The Oldest-Old

The number of adults aged 85 and over will rise from 3.3 million in 1994 to 8.6 million of the population by 2030, and to 19 million by 2050. It is this oldest-old cohort that represents a vulnerable population at risk for increased use of both acute and long-term care services. The oldest old have the highest rates of disability, nursing home use, and multiple chronic conditions. Average annual health expenditures for persons over age 65 are about 3.5 times greater than for persons aged 19–64, but for persons over age 85, they are almost six times greater.

As more people live longer and become the oldest-old, there may also be more who will experience chronic, limiting conditions or illnesses such as osteoporosis, arthritis, diabetes, dementia, heart disease or stroke. These are conditions in which individuals may become dependent on others for help in activities of daily living. In 1990–1991, the percentage of persons in the community dwelling population needing personal assistance with activities of daily living increased with age. Nine percent of the 65–69 year old cohort needed assistance while 50% of the elderly 85 and over needed personal assistance.

Given the growth of the aging population, especially the oldest with multiple chronic illnesses, the need for intermittent or continuous long term care services is growing. In 1980, 1.5 million older adults resided in nursing facilities and 4.5 million older adults received long term care services in their homes and communities; by the year 2000, two million will be in nursing facilities and seven million will require home and community-based long term care.

Responding to the Health Care Needs of Aging Americans

Although many older adults are healthy and functionally independent, a number will have high rates of physical and emotional disorders. As an example, the elderly have high rates of depression, suicide, anxiety, alcohol and drug abuse. The National Institute of Mental Health epidemiologic catchment area surveys indicate that these rates in the elderly today are only about one-fourth to one-third of those projected for the baby boomers as they become older adults.

These complex problems create a population of elders vulnerable to losing their ability to function independently and that are at risk of living with frailty. The nature of the needs of this increasing number of older people pose challenges for health care providers. Beyond acute, episodic health problems, the older person may have multiple, chronic health problems, interacting with social, emotional and environmental concerns. The health status of the elderly is also influenced by the many diverse cultural and ethnic backgrounds that characterize this population. Minority elders have higher rates of functional impairment, poverty, poor education, and malnutrition and have greater difficulty negotiating the health care system because of language and cultural barriers.

The needs of older adults, especially the frail or impaired, require a health care workforce knowledgeable about the systems and services of care with which the elderly interact, and the skill to provide care within these systems. Care of the elderly within managed care and long term care systems require a unique body of knowledge and practice. A working knowledge of case/care management as well as the ability to work cooperatively with case/care managers is necessary to be able to work cooperatively with managers. The ability to provide culturally competent geriatric health care requires a comprehensive fund of knowledge and cross-cultural geriatric training in community-based education. The complexity of problems common to older adults often demand the knowledge and skills beyond that of individual practitioners. Education is required to understand the principles of interdisciplinary teams and when they are appropriate to convene. Health promotion and disease prevention for older adults provide long term benefits for an aging population. These competencies must be learned.

A 1992 report by the Bureau of Health Professions notes that Federally sponsored studies and reports of the previous five years have consistently portrayed the health professions as unequipped to meet the present and future health care needs of older Americans. With few exceptions, health professions' faculty are not prepared to teach geriatrics and gerontology; curricula of basic and graduate level education do not include aging content; limited discipline-specific aging research is being conducted; and few health care professionals are choosing to care for the elderly. Little reward, professional or financial, is being given to those who care for the elderly. These obstacles will have far-reaching effects in the near future, when it is proposed that as much as two-thirds of a health care professional's time may be devoted to care of the elderly. A health workforce prepared with the knowledge base and technical skills of geriatrics and gerontology can respond more effectively and efficiently to the needs that arise from the challenges faced with advancing age. Through research, education and training, a skilled workforce can help reduce disability and functional limitations, improve the quality of life for both the aged and their loved ones, and can be an effective means of providing appropriate health care to an aging society. Further, there are cost-savings potentials of geriatrically prepared personnel, whose training would equip them to apply appropriate interventions (proper diagnosis, appropriate management, proper medications, use of assistive devices, and prevention approach to problem behaviors) that can forestall need for high-tech, high cost treatment.

The following chapters provide 1) critical reviews of the state of geriatric education within a rapidly changing health care environment and 2) policy recommendations to prepare the health workforce to meet the demands of an aging nation. A fundamental assumption in this text is that health professionals are colleagues working collaboratively in service to the elderly. Rehabilitative and respiratory therapists, psychologists, psychiatrists, and other mental health workers, nurses, social workers, dieticians, ethicists, dentists, physicians and other primary care providers, and the many additional disciplines reflected in the following chapters are partners in provision of care. The text provides a continuous quality improvement approach to the geriatric preparation of the health workforce. Contained within it are the educational seeds for a new generation of health care providers serving an aging nation.

Notes

Bureau of Health Professions Response. Shortage of Health Professionals Caring for the Elderly: Recommendations for Change. A report by the Chairman of the Select Committee on Aging, House of Representatives. December, 1992. Publication No. 102–915. U.S. Government Printing Office, Washington: 1993

Fowles, DC. A Profile of Older Americans. Washington DC: AARP, 1990.

Irvin, K, Riley, T, Booth, M, Fuller, E. Managed care for the elderly: A profile of current initiatives. Portland, ME: National Academy for State health Policy, 1993.

Manton, KG, Soldo, BJ. Dynamics of health changes in the oldest old: new perspectives and evidence. Milbank Memorial Fund Qtrly 1985; 63:2.

Sixty-five plus in the United States. Bureau of the Census Statistical Brief, SB/95/8, U.S. Department of Commerce, Economics and Statistics Administration, Bureau of the Census. Issued May, 1995.

U.S. Senate, Special Committee on Aging. Aging America, Trends and Projections. Washington, DC: U.S. DHHS. 1991.

1

Nursing

Kathleen Buckwalter, Pricilla Ebersole, Terry T. Fulmer, Joan B. McDowell, Ann L. Wall, May L. Wykle

THE STATE OF THE ART OF GERIATRIC NURSING EDUCATION AND TRAINING

Overview

In 1993, The Bureau of Health Professions (BHPr) published a Vision Statement which addressed health professions reform for the next century. The goal of BHPr, to improve the health status of Americans in the next century by enhancing education, utilization, distribution, and the quality of the nation's health personnel, was addressed via a strategic plan. Gerontological nursing must address these same areas if it is to meet the needs of older Americans. The discussion in this chapter relates to improvement in the quality and quantity of data concerning older adults and geriatric health care providers, the needs of special populations, research and related support issues, additional programs for geriatric specialists, reimbursement issues, and changes needed in nursing education. Past history and current situations are reviewed including problem areas, and recommendations are made for gerontological nursing education in the next century.

The Genesis and Trajectory of Contemporary Gerontological Nursing

As early as 1904, the American Journal of Nursing published an article on old age and disease. However, it was not until 1966, in response to the graying of the population, that the American Nurses Association (ANA) formed a Division of Geriatric Nursing, and not until 1970 that it developed and published the Standards of Geriatric Nursing Practice. In 1976 the ANA's Division of Geriatric Nursing was renamed the Gerontological Nursing Division to more accurately reflect the broad role nurses play in the management of the elderly.[1] In this document the terms "geriatric nursing," "gerontological nursing," and "gerontic nursing" are used interchangeably.

In the mid-seventies, graduate nursing programs throughout the United States began offering clinical specialties in gerontological nursing, several universities offered certificates in gerontological nursing and both certificate and graduate programs for geriatric nurse practitioners became available in several universities. Some of the pioneer educational programs that were begun included Cornell's PRIMEX geriatric nurse practitioner training program, the University of Colorado's and the State University of New York's certificate geriatric nurse practitioner programs, and Duke University's graduate geriatric nurse practitioner program. Educational opportunities in geropsychiatric nursing specialties did not develop until 1983, when the first geropsychiatric nursing program was offered at the Frances Payne Bolton School of Nursing at Case Western Reserve University through the support of a Special Projects Grant from the Division of Nursing.

Geriatric nursing has made substantial and impressive progress in the 25 years since the American Nurses Association first formally recognized the need for special emphasis on the care of the aged. In 1987 the ANA Gerontological Nursing Practice Standards refined the practice scope definition of the gerontological nurse as either a generalist or a specialist. The generalist functions in a variety of settings and draws upon the expertise of the specialist. The specialist requires a minimum of a master's degree in gerontological nursing.[2] Gerontological nurses are primary care and front line providers, both as specialists and generalists. As such, these nurses are most appropriate for coordinating and managing the care of the aged. Nursing is largely focused on health promotion, disease prevention, and long-term management of chronic disorders and their exacerbations which require prompt and intensive interventions.

Nurses can be proud of their long history as leaders in public health and home care nursing for in these areas they addressed many needs of elders. In these roles nurses pioneered new concepts such as case management and critical pathways. The role of the geriatric nurse in primary and managed care can best be described as that of the health care provider who assesses the clients' needs and strengths on an ongoing basis, who provides continuity of care, and referrals to appropriate health professionals and agencies, as well as coordination of the clients' total care.

Issues of Supply and Distribution

ANA data[3] show that only 6.6% of RNs are employed in nursing homes and extended care facilities, while 68% are employed in hospitals. Because of mergers, downsizing, and the use of trained technicians for numerous activities previously in the domain of RNs, the shift to use non-licensed personnel has resulted in a severe reduction of RNs in some settings. However, due to the intensity of care in acute care settings, the ratio of RNs to patients is now nearing 1:1. During the 1980's, due to the growing complexity and expanded responsibilities of nurses,[4] the ratio of RNs to patients increased from 77 nurses per 100 patients in 1982, to 99 per 100 in 1989.

In a recent assessment of the adequacy of health care personnel in various states, the U.S. Department of Health and Human Services (USDHHS) identified four occupations that most frequently posed supply problems: registered nurses, primary care practitioners, physical therapists, and licensed practical nurses.[5] Twenty-eight states identified particular needs for RNs, primary care practitioners, physical therapists, and LPNs; 41 of 52 states were concerned about the deficits in rural health care providers. A subsequent USDHHS study,[6] identified a shortage of almost

50,000 nurses in non-metropolitan areas of the United States. Forty-one states experienced great problems meeting the health needs of rural residents.[7] Shortages in these areas disproportionately affect the aged, because they tend to experience higher rates of chronic illness and disability and they are overly concentrated in rural populations.[9]

The Role and Influence of the Bureau of Health Professions

The Bureau of Health Professions has been described historically earlier in this document, and has had a major role in the development of educational opportunities for gerontological nursing. The following section describes special sections and programs within the BHPr.

The Division of Nursing

Since 1976, the Division of Nursing has funded 141 Advanced Nurse Education Programs at a cost of $17 million in an effort to develop educational programs with a specialty focus on gerontologic nursing. This has been made possible through Title VIII of the U.S. Public Health Service Act (PHSA). There are now nearly 50,000 nurse practitioners. More than half of these are certified, but only 1,572 are certified as geriatric nurse practitioners (GNPs). Although there are 58,000 clinical nurse specialists, only 493 are certified as geriatric clinical nurse specialists (GCNSs) which likely reflect the recency of a specific certification examination for geriatric clinical nurse specialists.[8] It is clear that many more nurses with geriatric specialty certification are needed.[9]

While the Division of Nursing has spent $67 million on professional nurse traineeships for GNPs and GCNSs since 1989, many positions are not available for nurses in areas where they are badly needed. For example, although there are 17,000 Medicare and Medicaid certified nursing homes in the United States, fewer than 700 certified nurse practitioners and/or clinical specialists are employed in these facilities.[10] As early as 20 years ago, Senator Daniel K. Inouye recommended that every nursing home over 100 beds should employ a geriatric nurse practitioner.[11] Clearly, there remains a great need for long-term care that is not being met. To compound this problem, federal support of the Division of Nursing's Special Projects Grants that have supported many of the training programs for geriatric nursing have been seriously curtailed.

Division of Associated, Dental and Public Health Professions

The United States federal government has played the most significant part in the development of geriatric nursing care as a specialized field of service. Through the support of Social Security Titles XVIII and XIX, the government mandated a program of care for the elderly before health care professionals had learned to do so. This mandate precipitated the rapid retooling of many care providers. To help with the retooling, the Division of Associated, Dental and Public Health Professions (DADPHP) has actively made resources and educational opportunities available to all of the numerous professionals who, by choice or necessity, have become specialists in the care of the aged. Through the support of Title VII of the PHSA, the DADPHP has supported a nationwide network of *Geriatric Education Centers* (GECs) since 1983. The GEC purpose is to provide education and training opportunities in geriatrics for health professions educators and practitioners. The Centers maintain resource clearinghouses and develop and disseminate curriculum and teaching materials. GEC materials pertinent to geriatric nurses include a wide range of audiovisual resources, bibliographies, curricular plans, systems of care, and topical foci such as stroke, falls, and elder abuse, as well as numerous other programs and study opportunities.

The Geriatric Education Centers have been particularly significant in the development of geriatric nurses. In the period between 1984 and 1993, 56,995 nurses were served by GEC training programs: 49,513 as participants in training programs with less than 40 hours and 7,482 as enrollees in programs with greater than 40 hours of training. Although interdisciplinary opportunities have been a highlight of the program offerings of the GECs nurses have been involved in GEC training programs to a greater extent than any other group of professionals. Of the more than quarter million trainees served by GECs in the decade from 1984 to 1993, nurses comprised over 20% of the total of all professionals participating.[12]

More to be Done: Special Populations

Long-Term-Care Needs

In the U.S. there are 53.3 long-term beds for every 1,000 seniors over the age of 65. There are 15,362 free standing facilities containing 1.7 million beds with for-profit nursing homes accounting for 74.5% of these facilities. The nursing home industry employs 1.3 million full-time and 368,000 part-time workers. Hospital sub-acute and long-term care beds accounted for another 92,000 beds. Average number of RNs per nursing home bed is 0.06; for profit homes have the lowest average of 0.05. Total employees per bed equal 0.88 with the highest percentage being Nurse's Aides (0.41).[13]

Difficulty recruiting and retaining qualified personnel to provide direct care in long-term care remains a critical problem. The major reason for the dearth of RNs in nursing homes is economic with federal and state regulations requiring very few RNs. In 1988 they received 88% of the typical acute care wage; by 1990 this percentage had dropped to 86%.[14] The five-year retention rate of nursing home nurses was 40%. Younger nurses have a lower retention rate of only 50% for one year while older nurses had a one year retention rate of 80%. The retention rate increased in concurrence with the increase in average weekly salary.[15] Typically, there is at least a $4 hourly discrepancy in pay with the nursing home nurse always on the short end.[15]

A 1992 USDHHS survey showed that the predominant employment site for RNs was the hospital. However, increasing numbers of hospital nurses were utilized in non inpatient bed units, such as out-patient departments, recovery rooms, and labor/delivery. Between 1980 and 1992, ambulatory care had the largest proportionate increase of registered nurses while between 1988 and 1992, the public/community health sector showed a large increase due to the number of nurses working in non-hospital-based home care agencies.

Minority Elders Needs

There is a growing number of minority elders and their caregivers living in underserved urban areas, where their economic plight and experience with discrimination affects health care. Nurse-managed clinics will be needed for geriatric outreach to this group as well as advanced gerontological nurse practitioners, clinical specialists, and geriatric mental health nurses. Minority elders need available gerontological services that are affordable, accessible, and culturally competent.

Rural Health Needs

Rural older adults represent a significantly underserved population. In many rural areas, nurses are the sole health care providers.[12] Geriatric nurse practitioners (GNPs) can provide primary health care services to older adults and consultation to families, as well as to personnel in home care and long-term care facilities. Because these advanced practice nurses can diagnose and manage common chronic and episodic health problems, they can help to promote, maintain, and restore health and maximize functional abilities. Geriatric nurse practitioners can effectively manage the majority of the common health problems experienced by geriatric patients[1] such as infections, congestive heart failure and arthritis.

Health Care for Older Women

Gynccological services for older women are often neglected. Recent studies have shown conclusively that, in spite of the great increase in breast cancer in older women and the Medicare cost coverage, these women are rarely directed to conduct routine breast self-exams or to obtain mammographies. Despite the fact that 45% of breast cancers are detected in women after age 65, only about 20% of older women have annual mammograms. Even in 1993, only 37% of care providers regularly recommended mammograms to their patients over 50 years of age.[14]

Urinary incontinence affects approximately 30% of elderly women.[16] Although nurses have been at the forefront of providing effective behavioral treatment for this common health problem as previously discussed, a majority of older women still do not have access to these services.[17] With greater emphasis on this problem and other women's health issues in the education of nurses, effective care of elderly women could become routine, resulting in reduced morbidity and improved functioning.

Needs of Elderly with Mental Health Problems

Although adults with mental health problems have traditionally been neglected in the U.S., advanced practice geropsychiatric nurses are establishing new models of care for mentally ill elderly. However, there is a great need for geropsychiatric advanced practice nurses to implement and provide care for the current unmet and projected future needs of the elderly. Increased funding for programs preparing geropsychiatric advance practice nurses would improve both the quantity and the quality of care for older adults with mental illness.

Another critical area for both graduate and undergraduate nursing is that of gerontological mental health. Currently, undergraduate psychiatric mental health experiences as well as graduate level programs, tend to underemphasize both gerontological mental health content and experiences. Anxiety, dementia, depression, substance abuse, plus all the traditional psychiatric mental health conditions are major concerns when caring for the elderly. Musil and Wykle[18] suggest that a minimal curricula content in nursing should address mental health promotion, cognitive disorders, psychiatric disorders, and substance abuse among the elderly. There are data that suggest that mental health problems in the elderly such as suicide and multiple missed diagnoses are much overlooked by all disciplines.

Scholarships, stipends and other financial inducements are needed to encourage nurse practitioners to practice with specific populations. Similarly, nurses from rural areas could be recruited to attend master's level nurse practitioner programs on conditional scholarships, getting their educational and living expenses paid only if they returned to their home areas or other rural settings to practice. These efforts would result in increased access to cost efficient quality primary health care for the rural elderly and their families.

International Nursing

As society moves rapidly into a global framework, it is incumbant upon the profession to think about key strategies for curricula that address multiple societies. international exchange programs which can assist the gerontological nurse to become accustomed to cultural diversity beyond this nation's framework is essential. As immigrants continue to enrich our culture, so too, they draw upon nursing resources across settings. Preemptive planning regarding gerontological nursing education and the global interface will place us in a competitve position going forward.

Information Systems

Given the historic evolution and numerous impinging social issues, one of the most critical tasks for government to perform for policy makers and educators is to develop a data bank that incorporates the numerous and often conflicting bits of information. For example, there should be one federal source of statistics that clearly identifies specific populations and their needs. It does not suffice to talk simply of "older adults." Within the forty-year span of time that is becoming the usual life expectation of "older adults," there are vast differences in needs, abilities and concerns. For example, the often quoted data regarding the increase of older adults in society reveals nothing about what needs they have, and whether or not these needs are being met. More reliable epidemiologic information is desperately needed if health professionals are to develop a true life span approach to the needs of the U.S. population. It is imperative that government agencies, health professionals, members of the business community, and private sector remain aware that the old of various ages are as different in their special care needs as are children from infancy to adolescence.

Future Projections and Visions

The fact that the numbers of older adults will continue to grow, and that the growth will be greatest for the old old population of elderly (i.e., 85 years plus), will have a great impact on future society and health care. Older persons use health care services at a higher rate than younger adults and the rate of utilization increases with age. Further, 1991 data showed an increase in out patient services by persons over age 65 and this trend is expected to continue. Preliminary data from a federal survey of 7,400 home health agencies in the U.S. showed that 74.5 percent of home care patients are 65 years of age and older.[19] Although hospital admissions and length of stay for the elderly has decreased since the implementation of Diagnostic Related Groups (DRGs), older persons continue to have a high rate of older persons admitted, even though chronically disabled or terminally ill younger patients are beginning to utilize these facilities at increasingly higher rates.

By 2030, the projected need for full time geriatric nurses in all settings is expected to reach 1.1 million. A 1989 study conducted by the American Academy of Nurse Practitioners revealed that 79 percent of family nurse practitioners (FNPs), 78 percent of adult nurse practitioners (ANPs), 99 percent of gerontological nurse practitioners (GNPs) and 42 percent of women's health nurse practitioners (WHNPs) cared for patients 65 years of age and older.[20] Those and other data included in this report clearly point to the need for increasing numbers of nurses with the knowledge and skills to provide quality primary health and chronic health care for aging adults.

To meet the needs of the growing number of elderly, the vision is that all basic nursing programs will include content regarding the health care of the older adults in their curriculums caring for adults; programs preparing adult and family nurse practitioners or clinical specialist will contain specific courses in geriatrics/gerontology for all students; additional geriatric specialists such as geriatric nurse practitioners (GNP) and clinical nurse specialist (CNS) are needed to provide chronic and primary care for the nation's elderly; and there must be nursing faculty prepared in geriatrics/gerontology in order to teach students. Efforts to encourage preparation of baccalaureate, masters and doctoral level faculty in geriatrics/gerontology is basic to accomplishing these goals. Mandating that students be taught by faculty prepared in geriatrics/gerontology will enhance learning and the quality of the finished product, the graduating student.

Education: The Mandate

Major efforts to educate nurses to provide quality elder care have produced many successes. These successes, however, cannot today produce the quantity or quality of nurses who are needed in the next century for adequate elder care. Gerontological nursing education must address certain key issues now if it is to meet these present and future challenges. The key issues are: model curricula; the use of advanced technology; increased interdisciplinary focus; adoption of standards for gerontological content; addressing existing curricular issues in relation to more geriatric content; state licensing issues; the need for continuing gerontological education; enrollment problems; and the need for geropsychiatric content.

Model gerontological nursing curricula have been proposed by numerous agencies both internal and external to nursing (e.g., ANA, NLN/Kellogg; Association for Gerontology in Higher Education; National Institute on Aging; Institute of Medicine; Pew). These agencies acknowledge that gerontological nursing is vital to elder care and has made a great contribution to this care. It is specifically because of this contribution, and the increasing need for gerontological nursing, that model curricula were proposed to address key issues in gerontological nursing education. These model criteria must now be used to assure needed gerontological content across levels of nursing education.

In the future, home care will use remote site technology and ethnocare specialists will be available to assist caregivers with culturally diverse populations. Managed care networks will also utilize this advanced communication technology to address quality assurance issues.

Interdisciplinary care that utilizes the latest communication technology will be necessary as the complexity of health care continues to increase and newer care delivery systems are designed. Ongoing cross-disciplinary consultation and collaboration, using both established as well as newer technologies such as fiber-optics, are needed for this care. Care will be inter-connected between primary care community centers, homes, and larger acute care facilities, linked via multiple modes of communication. Long distance, instantaneous consultation between interdisciplinary colleagues at multiple sites will be needed for delivery of quality elder care to large numbers living in both rural and urban settings.

All levels of gerontological education within nursing must contain interdisciplinary focused didactic content and clinical experiences. Mezey[21] pointed out that gerontological practice for all disciplines essentially takes place within an interdisciplinary milieu. The complicated nature of elder care requires both now and in the future, the assistance and interaction of many interdisciplinary colleagues. Nurses need to work with, for example, nursing assistants, social workers, physical therapists, pharmacists, physicians, health care administrators and many others in the provision of comprehensive elder care. Assessment and treatment data from specific disciplines needs to be considered in an open, collegial manner. Interdisciplinary teams in the future will be led not by a specific discipline, but by persons best prepared to coordinate such care.

Curricular standards in nursing were first addressed in the early part of the century, (NLNE, 1917, 1927, 1937), when the elderly comprised only a very small portion of the population; thus, gerontology content was not included in the early standards. As the population grew older, however, nursing began to focus more on older adults. Today many organizations have proposed criteria for gerontological nursing content in nursing curricula. These organizations include: the American Nurses Association (1994), the National League for Nursing with the Kellogg Foundation (1990), the Association for Gerontology in Higher Education (1990), and the National Organization of Nurse Practitioner Faculties (1993).

Since mid-century, nursing has experienced a swift development of its knowledge base that has led, in turn to a redefining of the domains and/or content areas within nursing. The current popular curricular structure—the three divisions of Chronic and Acute Care, Health Promotion and Disease Prevention, and Nursing Systems—are very different from past traditional areas such as medical surgical or pediatric nursing.

Model curricula and the standards suggested for gerontological content are, at times, in conflict with newer curricular ideals within the nursing profession. One potential conflict between model curricula and newer curricular designs concerns where to place gerontology content. Although this conflict is often discussed regarding graduate programs, there are counterpart discussions at all levels of the nursing curriculum. One approach which holds considerable promise is to present gerontological content via the use of expert "Master" gerontological faculty, who co-teach gerontological content as themes across all divisions and levels of the curricula. This approach is the opposite of positioning gerontological nursing content only within, for example, the division of Chronic Care. When gerontological nursing is not taught across all graduate programs, i.e., is situated only within one division, the gerontological content is inadequate.

A related curricular issue is whether to consider gerontological nursing a specialty or as part of primary care and other nursing programs. Factors driving this discussion are the realization that by the turn of the century, approximately 46% of all registered nurses will give direct care to elderly persons.[22] Although low student enrollment has consistently been a problem in advanced practice gerontological programs such as those of Gerontological Clinical Nurse Specialist and Gerontological Nurse Practitioner (i.e., the specialty areas), enrollments are increasing in primary care and other advanced practice programs in nursing. One suggested resolution is to provide gerontological nursing as both a specialty (which produces advanced practice clinical experts who demonstrate and give elder care and who act as consultants) and as a minor within primary care and other advanced practice nursing programs.

Undergraduate (both baccalaureate and associate degree) levels should also be addressed in model curricula. Many undergraduate programs have no separate undergraduate gerontology courses, a situation which has repeatedly been related to low gerontological nursing graduate enrollments, few faculty prepared in gerontology, and a lack of acceptance of gerontology content by nursing faculty. The introduction of undergraduate nursing content both separately as well as integrated throughout the undergraduate curriculum is necessary to prepare competent graduates. Undergraduate students must be cognizant of the aging process and of the developmental tasks confronted by elders as well as of their role in keeping elders functionally independent. Model curricula suggest that undergraduate education should consist of both didactic and clinical experiences with elderly persons in a variety of care environments. Although there have been many arguments against using nursing homes for placement of undergraduate students, newer trends in nursing home care may pre-empt many of these objections. Nursing homes currently and in the future will care for persons of all ages with an ever increasing level of acuity. Moreover, rehabilitation of persons of all ages will increasingly be addressed in nursing homes.

Nursing curricula also need to use and include more fully newer sites of care. In future health care, managed care delivery systems will likely use nursing homes as a mainstay for community primary care for the elderly. Chronic health conditions, once the major part of nursing home care, will continue to be addressed in nursing homes, although the tendency for acute settings to discharge all patients early will result in nursing homes serving as continuing care facilities for patients of all ages and at all levels of acuity. These factors all may result in nursing homes serving as an ideal placement for both students and faculty who wish to learn and update their knowledge of elder care.

Current state board examinations contain a surprisingly small proportion of gerontological nursing questions, particularly when compared to the large numbers of elders that nurses will serve in the next century. This situation tends to de-emphasize the need for gerontological content at the undergraduate level. One way to remedy this imbalance is to have nurses with current gerontological nursing preparation work with state boards to develop appropriate numbers and types of questions for these examinations. Another suggestion is to have faculty who are prepared as experts in gerontological nursing serve as master teachers and team-teach gerontology content with less prepared faculty. This team-teaching with master teachers tends to increase the acceptance of gerontology content within the overall curriculum; it also helps prepare additional numbers of gerontology faculty, using an adult education model.

Continuing Education

Continuing education in gerontological nursing should be a required component for relicensure. Many of the nurses caring for older adults have had little or no preparation in geriatrics. Yet these nurses have more frequent and intense patient contact than do other health care providers. In order to provide primary and chronic health care services of high quality, these nurses must be provided relevant and up-to-date continuing educational experiences. Continuing education of nurses to teach gerontological nursing content within all levels of the curriculum must also be addressed. Mid-career training of faculty is an essential mechanism for retooling individuals who have previously not been prepared for elder care nursing. Opportunities for these faculty to collaborate with neurological nurse specialists, cardiovascular nurse specialists, and others, are readily available. Every effort should be made to engage other faculty in gerontological nursing study. Examples such as the John A. Hartford Mid-Career Fellowship for Geriatric Medicine, or the NIMH Geriatric Mental Health Academic Award, can also be modeled within nursing.

The geriatric education centers (GECs), in existence since 1983, provide a ready conduit for the preparation of faculty who do not wish to repeat a graduate degree but still want intensive geriatric education and training. GEC programs, which have been successful in providing education for future nurses and other health care providers can serve as models for the expansion of GECs in each state. The outcome would be better geriatrically prepared nurses and other health care providers who have the knowledge and skills essential to provide quality care for this country's growing number of aging citizens.

Many University Centers on Aging offer graduate certificate programs. These programs provide graduate credits ranging from 12–20 or more that entitle students at both undergraduate and graduate levels to earn a certificate in gerontology. This allows nurses and faculty who are generalists or who specialize in areas other than gerontology to have a knowledge base for work with older adults.

Preparation of Nurses for Future Advanced Practice Roles

Dramatic shifts are also taking place within the acute care delivery system which relate to community care. The closing of acute care facilities across the nation, which is occurring at an even quickening pace, appears to be most severe in selected states such as California and Florida. These closures are changing dramatically the health care delivery system for elders, as nursing is moving more and more frequently into community based care.

A majority of community-dwelling older adults will continue to receive the bulk of their care in non-geriatric settings by non-geriatric specialists. Almost all managed care systems are based on the concept of a primary care practitioner coordinating and providing a majority of care for patients in the system, will ensure this situation or scenario. Therefore, greater emphasis must be placed on providing all nurses in advanced practice with didactic and clinical educational experiences in the care of the elderly. Because the educational programs that prepare nurse practitioners place such strong emphasis on the promotion of healthy life styles, the prevention of disease, and the maintenance and functioning of health, NPs are well suited for their role as primary care providers. In order to better utilize family and adult nurse practitioners in the care of the elderly, geriatric clinical and didactic courses must be provided for advanced practice nursing students. This will result in better care for the elderly regardless of which managed program or practice site an older person receives their care.

Congregate care, such as adult day care, is usually part of a managed care network, which may pose a coverage problem for elders who are increasingly mobile in their living arrangements. Although such care is often viewed in a positive light by elders due to their wish to receive care close to home, the increasing demand for a variety of types of community care will result in the need for increased numbers of nurses with geriatric preparation at the baccalaureate level and beyond. Interdisciplinary consultation must be available on a 24-hour basis across sites. Much of this technology is currently in place; nurse educators, however, need to be able to teach and model high-tech interdisciplinary consultation and to connect this high-tech care with nursing's traditional, personalized, caring approach.

Gerontological nursing education at the master's level has produced excellent advanced practice clinicians over the past three decades; these advanced practice nurses will deliver much of the primary care to elders via nurse-run clinics in the century to come.[23] Advanced practice nurses have demonstrated their skill as well as cost effectiveness across a variety of settings.[21] The Pew Commission[13] strongly suggests that advanced practice nurses will be a mainstay in newer health care delivery systems, such as managed care networks in the next century. Advanced practitioners, both GCNSs and GNPs, will join nurses with advanced preparation in primary care and other areas to provide elder care in both urban and rural settings. Nurse-run clinics—including those that are freestanding, those serving retirement communities, and those in nursing homes—enjoy great acceptance by the elderly. Thus advanced practice nurses will likely serve as a mainstay of care along with a cadre of other disciplines, in providing high quality interdisciplinary care to elders in ambulatory, long term care and acute care settings.

Reimbursement for Advanced Practice

The greatest impediment to advanced practice and the access of the elderly to quality primary and chronic care, delivered by nurses, is the lack of reimbursement. Nurse practitioners have demonstrated their ability to manage effectively and efficiently the majority of health problems that occur among elderly patients.[1] However, reimbursement for care has been an uphill battle. If improving the health and the quality of life for older adults is a major public health objective, then reimbursement for NPs should be a primary goal. Access to health care would be expanded and the quality of service enhanced if reimbursement for services were insured. To achieve this objective, federal agencies such as the BHPr and HCFA should support nursing organizations in their efforts to obtain legislation for reimbursement for the care nurses are now and will be providing for older adults.

Like geriatric medical fellowships, low enrollments in gerontological nursing masters programs have been a concern for both educational administrators as well as the health care industry in general. Several innovative attempts to increase the numbers of masters prepared gerontological nursing specialists, such as evening and weekend programs, have been somewhat successful. However, the numbers of specialists who will be needed in the future to serve in community care settings, to serve the rural elderly, and to serve their elderly in underserved, low economic areas, likely cannot be produced by current enrollments. Suggestions to produce the needed numbers of nurses and nurse faculty via these programs include the use of gerontological nurse master faculty to co-teach with faculty not so prepared, and the offering of gerontology as a minor in other advanced practice programs within nursing. In 1991 the American Nurses Association merged the councils of gerontological nursing CNSs and GNPs, but both types of specialists will be needed to care for the elderly.

Special Considerations for Graduate Programs

Research Support

Over the past ten years, knowledge regarding the aging process and the heterogeneity of older adults, as well as their special needs and strengths, has made geriatrics a viable area of study and clinical practice. Since many of the geriatric syndromes and problems have been issues traditionally managed by nurses, it is not surprising that much of the research in these area has been performed by nurse researchers and that findings from many of these studies are being incorporated into the practice setting. For example, nursing research focused on urinary incontinence[24, 25, 26] has led to the establishment of several nurse-managed continence programs for older persons. Most of these programs emphasize non-invasive, cost-efficient behavioral techniques. Thus, many older adults are now being successfully treated with bladder retraining, pelvic muscle exercises, and other behavioral modalities which are decreasing the use of pads, skin breakdown, and social isolation, while enhancing the quality of life. Studies of Strumpf and colleagues[27, 28] on restraints and falls have had a major impact on nursing care in long-term care facilities. Research showing that restraints cause more harm than good has unshackled numerous elderly and improved the quality of life of both hospitalized and nursing home residents.

A discussion of the state of the science of gerontological nursing education would not be complete without recognition of the role that nursing doctoral programs play in producing gerontological research. This research has had phenomenal growth as it addresses basic, applied, and clinical nursing questions. Geriatric nursing research, often rooted in nursing care problems and development of the basic science needed to address these problems, has gained wide acceptance in the scientific community in the last decades. Gerontological nurse researchers now sit on and chair many research review panels across various institutes. One way to continue this forward momentum of gerontological nursing research is to have certain doctoral programs focused specifically upon the needs of elders. There are several nursing doctoral programs which do so at the present time, but given the demographics of the future, more programs will need this focus.

Additional financial support for gerontological nursing research is needed. Gerontology and other nurse researchers in developmental stages of their careers should be provided fellowships with established researchers either to shift or upgrade to a gerontological focus in their research. Although there are a number of gerontological nurse researchers, their numbers are small and a number of critical issues such as geropsychiatric and health promotion needs of elders are not being addressed.

Several private foundations (e.g., Robert Wood Johnson, the Retirement Research Foundation) as well as federal agencies (e.g., NIA, NINR, NIMH, AoA, AHCPR, NIAMS) have attempted to address the need for greater levels of funding for gerontology nursing research, but the funds are still greatly limited and gerontological nurse researchers have not been supported in sufficient numbers. This situation is particularly unfortunate as the relationship between gerontological nursing practice issues and nursing research should be a dynamic one, with each informing the other.

Nursing research efforts are needed also to form the base for health care reform; new health care delivery efforts for the elderly must be evaluated both as to processes and outcomes. A strong knowledge base is also essential if gerontological nurses and others are to design and refine care for elders in the new health care delivery systems. Research initiatives for the development of home, nursing home, and community based health care are imperative, if efforts are to be of the quality required. Longitudinal and health care systems research is required to estimate the intended and unintended consequences of the newer and future health care delivery systems.

A number of private foundations and federal agencies listed above have portfolios related to aging research and regularly issue RFAs (Request for Applications) of interest to geriatric nurse researchers. It is essential that Congress ensure that these monies continue to be available for geriatric research efforts. However, the competition for successfully competing for NIH monies in aging-related research is daunting. Because of growing competition among investigators and decreasing pay lines, now commonly below 150. In many cases the quality of the proposals submitted by geriatric nurses need improved methodological rigor. This situation is particularly unfortunate in that the relationship between education, research and practice should be a dynamic one with research informing practice and teaching and with more curricula being research driven. Funding for research in a variety of venues including basic science, clinical trials, and longitudinal epidemiologic population-based studies related to nursing are all greatly needed.

Recent efforts at health care reform have stimulated interest in community based long-term care (CBLTC), an underdeveloped aspect of the current health care system. A strong knowledge base is essential if geriatric nurses and other providers are to contribute to the design and refinement of service delivery systems. So, too, are significant research funds from federal sources needed in order to conduct service delivery research that is needed for planning and evaluation purposes. Federal research and demonstration initiatives for the development of home and community based long-term care in the U.S. have contributed enormously to the development in the field to date, including state-level demonstrations and demonstrations such as Social health maintenance organizations, and On Lok, a CBLTC system in San Francisco, that have linked medical care and home care. But the knowledge base for further development is still inadequate, and more funding is needed to aid in the development and evaluation of state-level programs and to standardize state data systems for purposes of comparative longitudinal studies.

Currently, no one federal agency with a budget to support significant ongoing research programs in this area (both intra and extramural) has a priority concern with service delivery issues in CBLTC. However, a number of federal agencies (e.g., AOA, NINR, NIA, AHCPR) have scattered interest in CBLTC. The Office of the Asst. Secretary for Planning and Evaluation in DHHS has strong interest in CBLTC issues, but lacks both a mandate and the budget to support major research in the area. The need for more federal support for research on service delivery issues in long-term care is widely recognized by education and research centers in aging, at a level currently available for clinical and biomedical research (Caro and Callahan, Long-Term Care Task Force, presented at GSA November 1994).

Summary

The above discussion of the strengths and weaknesses found in the history of gerontological nursing in general and of gerontological nursing education in particular, leads to several recommendations. These recommendations, with their comprehensive statement or the action plan that must be addressed if gerontological nursing is to be effective in the next century. Likewise, if gerontological nursing education is to prepare the quantity and quality of nurses that are needed to meet the needs of the population it seeks to serve, each of the topics and their action plans must be taken seriously and addressed systematically.

The recommendations set forth in the next section flow logically from the information presented and their implementation is essential for gerontological nursing education to flourish and produce the required graduates in the next century. These recommendations are listed in a progression that is meant to indicate the interrelatedness of each. They are to be viewed as a composite; as a set, rather than individual recommendations.

RECOMMENDATIONS

Model Geriatric Nursing Curricula

1. Adaptation of model geriatric nursing curricula at both undergraduate and graduate levels.

Rationale

A number of model geriatric nursing curricula are currently available. For nursing to prepare sufficient numbers of expert gerontological clinicians, these curricula must be implemented at all educational levels and regularly evaluated to ensure that they meet minimal or exceed standards.

Action Required

1) Have accrediting agencies and organizations require schools of nursing to adopt one of the currently available model geriatric nursing curricula.
2) Have the BHPr support curricular consultation and evaluation efforts.
3) Gerontological nursing content must be offered as both a major and a minor, as a specialty in gerontological nursing master's programs, and as a minor in other advanced practice nursing programs. All these programs should include content on mental health, elder abuse, acute care, long term care and content on minority and rural aging.
4) Further, gerontological content should be freed from the confines of divisional structure (i.e., housed exclusively in the Division of Chronic Care). The result will be improved geriatric nursing education; standardized curricula which is readily disseminated via technology and delivered in innovative ways at both undergraduate and graduate levels. Gerontological nursing will be available as both a major and a minor in graduate nursing programs. More nurses will thus be prepared in gerontological and geropsychiatric

nursing, and elder Americans will be more likely to receive care from nurses with specific preparation in gerontological nursing, either in a primary care or specialist position. Nurses who are skilled in the use of advanced information technologies will be better positioned to provide care to elders in remote sites.

Responsible Agents

1) NLN, American Nurses' Association (ANA) and regional accrediting bodies,
2) BHPr,
3) Deans and
4) Faculty of Schools of Nursing.

Expected Outcomes

100% of all nursing programs in the country will have a gerontological curriculum in place within the next 5 years.

Undergraduate Gerontological Nursing Course

2. Implement freestanding undergraduate gerontological nursing courses that are available to all undergraduate students.

Rationale

This recommendation emerges from the need to meet the demand for more nurses with adequate geriatric knowledge.

Action Required

Have the accreditation bodies in nursing first recommend, and by the year 2000 require, a separate undergraduate gerontological nursing course for all nursing programs.

Responsible Agents

NLN, ANA and other accrediting bodies, Deans and Faculty of Schools of Nursing.

Expected Outcome

All basic nursing programs in the United States will have core content in gerontological nursing in 3 years.

State of the Art Technology in Gerontological Teaching Endeavors

3. All programs should set goals related to phasing in and enriching the information technology strategies throughout the curricula.

Rationale

State of the art informatics and technology should be the basis from which these curricula are generated, and will set the stage for enhanced collaboration across sites and programs. Advanced information technologies (i.e., fiber optic and digital networks) will increasingly be used in homes, nursing homes, nurse-run clinics, and other systems of care. Many elders reside in remote urban and rural settings, and nurses will need to be proficient in the use of instruments such as the fiber optic otoscope, television telephones, and other monitoring and data transfer devices, in order to provide care to these elders in future health care delivery systems.

Action Required

1) Those schools with expert faculty in geriatrics and advanced technologies and with model curricula already in place should provide consultation, curricular materials, etc. to schools of nursing which desire to implement geriatric nursing training and curricula featuring knowledge of advanced technologies.
2) Incorporate advanced technologies, such as long distance assessment and management of care using laser transfer of data and joint consultation at remote sites.

Responsible Agents

1) The Schools of Nursing working with the National Library of Medicine, (NLM)
2) The computer science and informatics sections at their respective institutions, and the
3) ANA.

Expected Outcome

100% of all programs will have informatics as a part of their teaching and learning strategies within the next 3 years.

Gerontological Masters Courses

4. Gerontological Masters Courses as electives or as basis of a minor to all graduate nursing students.

Rationale

The paucity of adequately prepared faculty in gerontological nursing and the difficulty with recruitment of students into the field set the stage for new ways of dealing with old problems. All graduate students should be encouraged to elect gerontological courses and it is encumbant upon the faculty to point out the relevance to practice in every conceivable nursing role. The "gerontologicalization" of graduate students can increase the number of knowledgeable students, who may, in turn, develop an interest if not a responsibility toward geriatric practice.

Action Required

1) The NLN should review language in the current documents for accreditation in order to address this action.
2) Graduate programs should be required to have a minimum of 1 course available for graduate students and for those programs that have graduate programs in gerontological nursing, they should be required to open those classes to all specialty students. Over 50 programs would be able to immediately implement this action.

Responsible Agent

1) NLN,
2) Graduate programs in Nursing.

Expected Outcome

An immediate increase in the number of master's prepared nurses with some base in gerontological nursing. In 5 years, 100% of this master's prepared workforce would be aware of and knowledgeable about basic issues in geriatric care.

State Board Examinations

5. Increase the number of geriatric and geropsychiatric questions on state board examinations.

Rationale

More geriatric-related questions on the licensing exam will support increased emphasis on geriatric content at the undergraduate level.

Action Required

Identify nursing faculty with expertise in gerontological nursing in each state to work with members of their state boards of nursing as item writers and content experts to enhance both the quality and quantity of geriatric and geropsychiatric questions on licensing exams.

Responsible Agents

State Boards of Nursing, National State Board Test Pool Office, Faculty of Schools of Nursing.

Expected Outcome

In 5 years, 20% of the questions on state licensing exams will include content related to geriatric and geropsychiatric content. This increased emphasis will help ensure that graduates from all nursing programs will be required to possess adequate gerontological nursing knowledge.

Continuing Education in Gerontological Nursing

6. Mandate continuing education credits in gerontological nursing for re-licensure.

Rationale

The pool of nurse educators and clinicians must continually update their knowledge base in gerontology. This recommendation is particularly important for nurses who graduated without receiving gerontological content as part of their training. Moreover, a precedent for required content for re-licensure has already been set in the areas of child abuse and universal precautions.

Action Required

1) Encourage expert geriatric nurses to work with state re-licensure agencies and continuing education departments to develop more relevant, current continuing education offerings in geriatrics.
2) These offerings should be made widely available through interesting and innovative methods of dissemination, i.e., telecommunication conferences.

Responsible Agents

1) State re-licensure boards, expert gerontological nurses,
2) Directors of departments of continuing education, GECs.

Expected Outcome

State Boards will require a minimum of 1 credit of gerontological nursing content for re-licensure in 3 years.

Traineeships for Faculty and Student Training in Gerontological Nursing and Research

7. Restore and expand traineeships for both gerontological nursing faculty and students at the master's through post-doctoral levels.

Rationale

Enhanced training opportunities for faculty and graduate students will increase the knowledge base that supports geriatric nursing practice and leads to higher quality gerontological nursing research. Traineeships should increase the number of nurses interested in and qualified to work with the elderly. Make special efforts to enroll minority nurses in such traineeships. Federal set-aside moneys should be earmarked for the development of minority faculty and advanced practice specialists in geriatric nursing. The increased availability of traineeships will increase the number of nurses with geriatric clinical and research expertise who are available to provide primary care to older, underserved Americans and to evaluate outcomes associated with that care.

Action Required

1) Set aside specific funds at the federal levelfor the preparation of gerontological nursing faculty and graduate students.
2) Professional Nurse Traineeships (Section 830) should be split into two subsections:
a) grants that are distributed to schools of nursing to use as they see fit, and
b) full tuition plus a stipend with a service payback in a facility working with the elderly.
3) Advanced Nurse Education (Section 821) should be redirected to post-master's and doctoral training to prepare new, or retrain existing faculty for clinical education

of advanced practice nurses.
4) In order to receive Advanced Nurse Education funds, trainees would be required to work with the underserved elderly for a minimum of two years following graduation.

Responsible Agents

1) U.S. Congress;
2–4) Division of Nursing.
Expected Outcome
50% increase in gerontological nursing traineeships in 3 years with a concomitant increase in the number of graduates.

Increased Numbers of Minorities in Gerontological Nursing

8. Provide increased incentives for minority nurses to enter gerontological nursing at the graduate level.

Rationale

Sociodemographic changes indicate an increasing number of minority elders in the U.S. More minority geriatric nurses prepared at advanced levels are needed to meet the needs of the growing, underserved minority population.

Action Required

1a) Make special efforts to enroll minority nurses in graduate programs such as targeted traineeships,
b) linkage programs with TBCUs (traditionally black colleges and universities.)
c) Outreach to high schools for minority students with stipends and tuition reimbursement.

Responsible Agents

BHPr, Schools of Nursing, Congress of the United States.

Expected Outcome

An increase of 20% in the number of minority graduates in 5 years.

Interdisciplinary Training and Consultation

9. Enhance interdisciplinary experiences at all levels of the geriatric nursing curriculum.

Rationale

Geriatric care in the next century will be increasingly interdisciplinary in nature. Students from a variety of disciplines should be exposed to interdisciplinary endeavors in their training if they are expected to practice in a cooperative, collegial manner following graduation. The provision of interdisciplinary training fellowships would be a major asset to such collegial development. More high quality, coordinated, and interdisciplinary care will be delivered to elders by interdisciplinary teams of health care professionals who have well-established processes of communication and interaction.

Actions Required

1) Support nursing curricula and basic medical education efforts to provide joint training and educational experiences in the assessment and management of older adults.
2) The federal government, in cooperation with private foundations, should provide new funds for 50 interdisciplinary training fellowships by the year 2000.

Responsible Agents

1) Faculty of Schools of Medicine and Nursing,
2) BHPr, private foundations such as John A. Hartford Foundation and Brookdale Foundation.

Expected Outcomes

50 interdisciplinary training fellowships in 5 years and 50% of the graduate programs would have implemented a model interdisciplinary course.

Compensation for Geriatric Nurses

10. Ensure adequate compensation for nurses who work with the elderly.

Rationale

Geriatric nurses, especially those working in long-term care settings, receive lower salaries than nurses in either acute care or home care settings. The inequity and lack of financial incentives has contributed to difficulties attracting and retaining qualified nurses in geriatrics and long-term care. Recruitment and retention of geriatric nurses, especially in long-term care settings, will be enhanced.

Actions Required

1) Encourage health care delivery organizations to increase RN compensation and improve their long-term career orientation.
2) Provide a one-time adjustment to raise RN relative wages, targeted to geographic and institutional differences in providing care to the elderly.
3) Develop and implement innovative options for nurses to choose and to remain in systems that provide care to the elderly.
4) Expand RN pay ranges based on experience, performance, education, and demonstrated leadership.

Responsible Agents

1) ANA,
2) HCFA,
3) Insurance agencies,
4) American Association of Homes for the Aged.

Expected Outcome

Equity in pay for all geriatric nurses in 5 years.

Improvement of the Quantity and Quality of Data Related to Older Adults Programs

11. Resolve conflicting reports regarding the current data related to older adults.

Rationale

Before any group can understand the current statuses, resources, and needs of aging Americans or make accurate predictions about their future requirements, a comprehensive, standardized data base is necessary. More accurate predictions of future needs of older Americans will be possible and planning for services and policies will be more logical and realistic.

Action Required

1) Establish a comprehensive, standardized data collection methodology under the auspices of one or two government agencies.
2) These agencies should update information related to health, economic, and social issues of older Americans on a periodic basis in order to document the present situation of the nation's heterogeneous aging population and to predict future educational needs more accurately.

Responsible Agents

1) USPHS,
2) Division of Nursing, National Institute on Aging.

Expected Outcome

A status report on data sources, quality, and gaps by 1999.

12. Improve the data related to geriatric nursing education and subsequent projections related to employment opportunities.

Rationale

Numerous and conflicting reports regarding the distribution and employment of nurses providing care for the elderly makes future planning for geriatric education requirements difficult. Data based on more precise terms, job descriptors, and definitions will allow educators, researchers, and policy makers to understand more about the care provided by geriatric nurses than possible with data under the current system, which reports information basically limited to the number of nurses working in various care settings. As in the prior recommendation, more accurate and comprehensive data will permit more realistic predictions of the future educational and practice needs of geriatric nurses.

Action Required

1) Develop a consensus among both government and private agencies on the definitions of terms such as "professional nurse," "geriatric education," and "geriatric prepared." In addition,
2) develop descriptors that accurately identify what geriatric nurses in various employment settings actually do (e.g., management, patient care activities) in order to provide more useful information.

Responsible Agents

1) Division of Nursing, Robert Wood Johnson Foundation.
2) National League for Nursing

Expected Outcome

A status report on gerontological nursing education produced in 3 years.

Increased Numbers of Nursing Faculty Prepared in Gerontological Nursing

13. Enhance opportunities for mid-career training of faculty to re-tool and obtain geriatric content through the provision of faculty development awards, fellowships, short term courses, certificate programs, continuing education offerings in geriatric nursing, and opportunities to work with master teachers in gerontology.

Rationale

Faculty who have learned geriatric skills and content are more likely to support the introduction of gerontological content in the curriculum and to improve the quality of education in both undergraduate and advanced practice programs. A critical mass of geriatric nurse educators will thus be developed and the pool of nursing faculty prepared in geriatric nursing will be increased.

Action Required

1) Provide education for faculty members not prepared in geriatric nursing by awarding two competitive faculty development awards annually, by supporting faculty attendance at GEC training programs, and by using approaches that have been successful in geriatric medicine such as the John A. Hartford Mid-Career Fellowship.
2) Release time must be provided by academic institutions so that faculty can achieve continuing education goals, such as attendance at GEC training programs. Faculty must design their own didactic and clinical experiences in time-limited programs.
3) Master teachers in gerontological nursing must work with unprepared faculty and co-teach gerontological nursing courses with them.

Responsible Agents

1) Bureau of Health Professions (BHPr), NIA, National Institute for Nursing Research (NINR), and the John A. Hartford Foundation,
2) Deans and
3) Faculty of Nursing Schools

Expected Outcome

In 5 years, 20% of all nursing faculty will have had geriatric education.

Geriatric Nursing Research Funding

14. Implement a number of assistive strategies including postdoctoral training opportunities, conferences, and grantsmanship and proposal development workshops, to enhance the ability of geriatric nurse researchers to obtain extramural research funding.

Rationale

Geriatric nursing research has directly benefitted older patients in terms of improving care practices and quality of life, and nurse scholars need to become more competitive in aging-related research funding. Improved proposals with greater methodologic rigor will merit consideration for funding. The relationship between education, research, and practice should be a dynamic one, with research informing practice and teaching and with more curricula being research-driven.

Action Required

1) Increase the number of post-doctoral opportunities in geriatric nursing to prepare future researchers;
2) fund annual "mini" consensus conferences (on different geriatric topics each year) with invited papers from experts in the field, from which a research agenda in geriatric nursing would be developed and RFAs and allocation of funds would follow;
3) encourage GECs and Centers on Aging to hold geriatric nursing faculty training workshops in grantsmanship and proposal development; and
4) have NIH agencies sponsor grant workshops that would include a competitive review of research ideas submitted by geriatric nurses in five-page "mini proposals." Ten to 15 proposals would be selected annually and the researchers invited to Washington, DC, for a two-day workshop staffed by NIH project officers (to teach the strategies of getting grants funded) and methodological experts (to critique proposed designs and data analysis ideas). The above actions should ensure that nurse researchers will be better prepared to compete successfully for funds to conduct geriatric studies that will enhance service delivery systems and the health of aging Americans. In particular, an increased number of geriatric nursing research proposals will be submitted to private foundations and the National Institutes of Health, and an increasing percentage of those proposals will receive fundable priority scores. More geriatric nurses will complete post-doctoral training, and more faculty will infuse research- based content into their geriatric curricula.

Responsible Agents

1–4) National Institute for Mental Health (NIMH), NIA,
2) NINR, Agency for Health Care Policy and Research (AHCPR), and Administration on Aging (AOA)
3) University Centers on Aging and GECs..

Expected Outcome

A ten-fold increase in funded nurse investigators over the next 5 years.

Funding for Geriatric Demonstration Projects Which Can Inform Nursing Education

15. Ensure that service delivery issues across settings including the home and CBLTC receive the national attention and support.

Rationale

Recent efforts at health care reform have stimulated interest in community-based long-term care (CBLTC), as well as other multidisciplinary delivery models. The underdeveloped aspects of the current health care system require focus to determine their respective merits. A strong knowledge base is essential if geriatric nurses and other providers are to contribute to the design and refinement of the service delivery system. So, too, are significant research funds from federal sources needed in order to conduct service delivery research that is needed for planning and evaluation purposes. Federal research and demonstration initiatives for the development of home and community based long-term care in the U.S. have contributed enormously to the development in the field to date. However, the knowledge base is still inadequate, and more funding is needed to help develop and evaluate state-level programs and to standardize state data systems for purposes of comparative longitudinal studies. The research will provide the basis for modifications in the current health care system as it expands and matures.

Action Required

Congressionally mandate intramural and extramural research programs with particular emphasis on the development of state programs and the dissemination of research findings.

Responsible Agents

Responsibility for the research program could be placed in an existing federal agency (e.g., AOA, NIA, Office of the Assistant Secretary for Planning and Evaluation at DHHS). Private foundations should be encouraged to provide seed money for development of the proposed program.

Expected Outcome

A 20-fold increase in the number of rigorously evaluated demonstration projects over the next 5 years.

Geriatric Nursing Education Related to Special Populations

16. Include didactic content and clinical experiences with diverse groups of older persons in geriatric nursing education.

Rationale

It is no longer relevant to discuss persons over 65 as a homogeneous group. Geriatric nursing education must recognize the specific characteristics and needs of various population groups in America such as: rural Americans, aging women, and older adults with mental health problems. Moreover, each minority group has a unique culture, with problems and strengths that need to be identified. Graduates will provide more culturally competent and sensitive geriatric care and attend to the unique needs and circumstances of the growing number of older minority adults and those with different health care problems as a result of such actions.

Action Required

1) Have geriatric nursing education programs (both undergraduate and graduate and continuing education) emphasize content on

cultural competence in their curricula, including didactic and clinical experiences with older persons from diverse cultures, socioeconomic groups, and geographic regions, and representing both genders. Geropsychiatric content and experiences with mentally ill older adults should also be included.
2) Accrediting bodies should require geriatric nursing education programs to include culturally competent content and experiences.

Responsible Agents

1) Division of Nursing, Faculty of Schools of Nursing.
2) NLN.

Expected Outcome

All programs will identify appropriate curricular content in 5 years to retain accreditation.

Education for Geriatric Nurses in Advanced Practice Roles

17. Support the education of geriatric clinical nurse specialists and geriatric nurse practitioners in the provision of direct care and lead other members of the health care team in delivering effective health care for older adults.

Rationale

GNSs and GNPs are needed to meet the varied and complex needs of the aging population through professional leadership, education of elders and professional nurses and direct care.

Action Required

Provide support and leadership, modelling the essential nature and differences of each role while placing them within the advanced practice framework emerging for the profession.

Responsible Agents

Faculty of Schools of Nursing, the ANA and other certifying agencies that influence nursing practice and role.

Expected Outcome

The number of masters prepared GNSs and GNPs will increase by 10% in 3 years.

Reimbursement for Advanced Practice Nurses

18. Reimburse master's and doctorally prepared advanced practice geriatric nurses (GNPs and GCNSs) by Medicaid and Medicare and other third-party payers for their clinical services.

Rationale

Access to health care is in part determined by the ability of health care providers to be reimbursed for their services. The Health Care Finance Committee and various legislators have supported the need for reimbursement for nurse practitioners, but their efforts have been stymied by powerful opposing lobbies. Advanced practice geriatric nurses must be recognized as valuable colleagues in the provision of effective, quality health care to elders, many of whom experience health care problems within the purview of nursing care (e.g., incontinence, falls, skin breakdown). More health care facilities will employ advanced practice geriatric nurses once they can be reimbursed for the care they provide in these facilities. This, in turn, should increase accessibility to care, especially for poor and underserved elders.

Action Required

Pass legislation that provides for Medicare, Medicaid, and other third-party payers (e.g.,

Blue Cross/Blue Shield) to reimburse advanced practice geriatric nurses for the health care services they provide.

Responsible Agents

U.S. Congress, Health Care Financing Administration.

Expected Outcome

Universal reimbursement for advanced practice geriatric nurses by 1998.

International Gerontological Nursing

19. Promote state-of the-art curricula related to international gerontological nursing that can be applied across nations

Rationale

As society moves rapidly into a global framework, it is incumbant upon the profession to think about key strategies for curricula that address multiple societies. International exchange programs which can assist the gerontological nurse to become accustomed to cultural diversity beyond this nation's framework are essential. As immigrants continue to enrich our culture, so too, they draw upon nursing resources across settings. Preemptive planning regarding gerontological nursing education and the global interface will place us in a competitve position going forward.

Action Required

Convene an international forum within the International Council of Nursing and /or Sigma Theta Tau to outline global issues related to gerontological nursing.

Responsible Agent

ICN and Sigma Theta Tau

Expected Outcomes

A white paper outlining key elements of an international gerontological nursing curricula in 2 years.

REFERENCES

1. Ebersole PE, Hess PA. Toward healthy aging: human needs and nursing response, 4th ed. St. Louis: Mosby, 1994.
2. American Nurses Association. Standards and scope of gerontological nursing practice. Kansas City, MO: American Nurses Association, 1987.
3. McKibbin RC. The nursing shortage and the 1990's, realities and remedies. Kansas City: American Nurses Association, 1990.
4. Pew Health Professions Commission. Health professions education for the future: school in service to the nation. San Francisco: Pew Health Professions Commission, 1993.
5. USDHHS. States' assessment of health personnel shortages: issues and concerns. Rockville, MD: Health Resources and Services Administration (DHHS No. HRS-P-OD 90-6), 1990.
6. USDHHS. The registered nurse population: findings from the national sample survey of registered nurses. Rockville, MD: USDHHS, Public Health Service, Bureau of Health Professions, March 1992.
7. USDHHS. Rural health professions facts: Supply and distribution of health professionals in rural America. (CB # 7590). Chapel Hill, NC, North Carolina Rural Health Research Program, University of North Carolina at Chapel Hill, 1992.
8. USDHHS. An agenda for health professions reform. Rockville, MD: USDHHS, Public Health Service, Bureau of Health Professions, 1993.
10. Health Resources and Services Administration. National employment estimates of selected health care personnel in home health

care agencies, hospices, nursing homes, board and care (residential) homes. Washington, DC: Health Resources and Services Administration, 1991.
11. Institute of Medicine. Nursing and nursing education: Public policies and private actions. Washington, DC: National Academy Press, 1983.
12. Bureau of Health Professions. Health resources and services administration. In shortage of health care professions caring for the elderly: recommendations for change. Washington, DC: U.S. Gov. Print Office (Comm. Pub. No. 102–915), 1993.
13. American Health Care Association. AHCA issue and data book for the United States Congress. Washington, DC: American Health Care Association, 1991.
14. USDHHS. Analysis of the environment for the recruitment and retention of registered nurses in nursing homes. Rockville, MD: Health Resources and Services Administration, 1987.
15. Health Care Compensations Services. A graphic comparison of registered and licensed practical nurses in nursing homes, home care agencies and hospitals. Oakland, New Jersey: HCS, 1994.
16. Diokno AC, Herzog AR, Brock BM, Brown MS. (1986). Prevalence of urinary incontinence and other urological symptoms in the non-institutionalized elderly. J Urology 1986; 136:1022–1025.
17. McDowell BJ, Silverman M, Martin D, Musa, D, Keane C. Identification and intervention for urinary incontinence by community physicians and geriatric assessment teams. J. Am Geri Soci 1994; 42:501–505.
18. Musil C, Wykle M. (in press). Psychiatric mental health content for gerontological nursing education. In T. Fulmer & MA Matzo (Eds.), *Strengthening Gerontological Nursing Education.* New York, N. Y.: Springer.
19. Straham, G. An overview of home health and hospice care patients: preliminary data from the 1993 National Home and Hospice Care Survey. Hyattsville, MD: National Center for Health Statistics (Publication No. 256), 1994.
20. Select Committee on Aging. Shortage of health care professionals caring for the elderly: recommendations for change. Washington, DC: U.S. Government Print Office (Comm. Pub. No. 102–915), 1993. 21. Mezey, M. Why good ideas have not gone far enough. Presentation at a Merck sponsored conference on 1/6/1994. N.Y., N.Y. (unpublished manuscript)
22. Wells T. Setting the agenda for GN. In Heine (Ed.), Determining the future of GN education. New York: N.L.N, 1993.
23. Pew Health Professions Commission. Healthy America: practitioners for 2005. Philadelphia: administered through Duke University Medical School, 1993.
24. Brink CA, Sampselle CM, Wells TJ, Diokno, AC, Gillis GL. A digital test for pelvic muscle strength in older women with urinary incontinence. Nur Res 1989; 38(4):196–199.
25. Wyman JF, Elswick RK, Wilson, MS, Fantl JA. Relationship of fluid intake to voluntary micturations and urinary incontinence in women. Neuro & Urodynamics 1991; 10:463–473.
26. Colling J, Ouslander J, Hadley BJ, Eish, J, Cambell, E. The effects of patterned urge-response toileting (PURT) on urinary incontinence among nursing home residents. J Am Geri Soci 1992; 40:135–141.
27. Strumpf NE, Evans LK, Schwartz D. Physical restraint of the elderly. In Clinical gerontological nursing: a guide to advanced practice. Philadelphia: W. B. Saunders, 1991.
28. Strumpf NE, Evans LK, Wagner J, Patterson J. Reducing physical restraints: Developing an educational program. J Gero Nur 1992; 18(11):21–27.

ACKNOWLEDGMENTS

The authors wish to thank Mr. Subash Sharma and Ms. Diane Ferris from the

Frances Payne Bolton School of Nursing for their technical assistance with the preparation of this manuscript, and Geraldine Felton, of the University of Iowa and Mathy Mezey of New York University for their editorial assistance.

2

Public Health

Ann H. Cary, Thomas Prohaska, Myrna Silverman, and Steven P. Wallace

THE STATE OF THE ART OF GERIATRIC PUBLIC HEALTH EDUCATION AND TRAINING

Introduction

Public health is unique among the health professions in its primary focus on populations rather than individuals, its specialization in protecting health rather than treating diseases, and its concern with the context within which health is maintained and promoted. This perspective is important for older populations as modern medicine reaches its limits in treating chronic illness and society increasingly looks towards prevention. As large numbers of older adults live to older ages, there will also be an increasing emphasis on maintaining functional independence and maximizing quality of life rather than extension of the average life expectancy. Public health is positioned to be especially useful in addressing prevention and quality of life issues. This expertise also encompasses skills and knowledge in the organization and financing of health care organizations and systems, promoting quality, adequacy, and equity as the profession attempts to improve the efficiency of the health care system. The growing importance of public health for older adults is placing increasing demands on a workforce that has limited training in public health and aging. If the health care infrastructure is to be adequate to face the health and aging issues of the next century, there is a compelling need to improve and expand the education and training of public health professionals in the area of public health and aging.

What is Public Health?

The roots of public health are in the sanitary movement of the 1800s, where the concern was with providing safe drinking water to prevent the outbreak of disease. During the following 100 years public health continued to focus especially on communicable disease. Because plagues and epidemics have been nearly eliminated as health problems in the industrialized world, the work of public health has shifted away from acute illness and towards chronic health problems and social conditions that create poor health. Some of the most visible public health programs currently include smoking control, violence prevention, teen pregnancy deferral, and AIDS prevention.

For older adults, public health has grown to encompass a wide range of programs, from "heart healthy" campaigns to Alzheimer's caregivers support programs to health insurance advocacy organizations. This range of activities can be described as involving three different levels of primary health care: (1) primary prevention that involves preventing health problems (classically through immunization programs; but also through health education, environmental protection, and policy development); (2) secondary prevention through the early identification and treatment of health problems (such as high blood pressure screening); (3) tertiary prevention which aims to ameliorate the consequences of disease and disability (such as through making buildings wheelchair accessible, organizing meals on wheels programs, or developing methods to improve the quality of care in nursing homes).

The application of central public health principles to older adults is well illustrated by the health promotion and disease prevention report, *Healthy People 2000*[1]. This report sets out health objectives for the nation, the majority of which require public health approaches to achieve. The three principle goals in that report are:

- increasing the span of *healthy* life,
- reducing health disparities, and
- achieving access to preventive services for all.

Almost one-third of the 298 specific objectives in that report are applicable to older individuals, covering items such as physical activity, nutrition, unintentional injuries, heart disease and stroke, cancer, and diabetes and chronic disabling conditions.[2] This ambitious set of objectives will also serve as the framework for health objectives well into the 21st century, and will create a continuing need for a well-trained workforce in public health and aging who can develop the needed programs and policies to achieve these goals, assure the adequacy and effectiveness of the programs, assess new and on-going health problems as targets for intervention.

As health care costs continue to rise in the United States and the population includes increasing numbers of older adults, the need for public health practitioners with training in aging will grow rapidly. The nation already faces a shortage of trained public health practitioners in general—it has been estimated that under half of all persons working in public health practice have formal training in public health.[3] This training is critical since public health is an interdisciplinary field, drawing on behavioral and social sciences, biostatistics, epidemiology, environmental health, and health policy and administration.

Public health is also a crucial link in the move towards strengthening primary care for aging persons in the country. The Pew Health Professions Commission[4] identifies seven key competencies for primary health practitioners, at least four of which involve central issues in public health education and practice. *Care for the Community's Health* entails the public health mission of population and health promotion/disease prevention foci when it calls for practitioner competency in integrating a range of activities that promote, protect and improve the health of the community. *Practice Prevention and Promote Healthy Lifestyles* is a competency grounded in public health research and practice in primary and secondary prevention. *Participate in the Emerging System and Accommodate Expanded Accountability* involves a multidisciplinary approach to health services delivery and involvement in health policy development that involve the health services component of public health. *Involve Patients and Families in the Decision-Making Process* requires the behavioral science base of public health, and that is reflected in many public health education programs. In addition, public health provides a bridging discipline that helps unite primary care specialties. Many physicians obtain public health degrees to enhance their skills in health administration, preventive health, and/or epidemiology. Public health and nursing have had an ambitious history together. Dentistry provides a successful example of how public health can work with a clinical discipline, and how clinical practice that incorporates principles of prevention can have a dramatic impact on health status. The interaction between pharmacy and public health in the past has been limited, but is bound to grow with the new push to have pharmacists also work as educators.[5] The relationships make public health a natural discipline to work with all health professions in the needed shift away from narrow disciplinary approaches to the health problems of the elderly and towards more interdisciplinary models.[6]

Public health education occurs in a variety of institutional arrangements. Training in the 27 Schools of Public Health provides comprehensive instruction in the five core areas of public health (behavioral and social science, biostatistics, environmental health, epidemiology, and health policy/administration). There are also 25 specialized programs that offer public health degrees outside of schools of public health, primarily in health education and departments of community health/preventive medicine. Schools and programs that offer professional degrees in public health (MPH and DrPH) are accredited by the Association of Schools of Public Health (ASPH). In addition, many schools of nursing offer a specialization in public health or community health nursing under the accreditation of the National League of Nurses (NLN). The term "accredited public health programs" and the recommendations in this chapter refer to the schools and programs offering degrees or specializations in public health that have specific accreditation standards that cover public health.

Public Health and Aging, Geriatrics, and Gerontology

This chapter addresses the education and training needs in "public health & aging" as a field related to, but distinct from geriatrics and gerontology. Geriatrics is typically understood to e a branch of medicine that deals with the problems and diseases of old age and aging people, with a particular focus on clinical interventions at an individual level.[7] The focus of public health on *prevention* and interventions at a *group level* distinguish public health and aging from geriatrics. Gerontology is an all-encompassing field that includes all scientific study of the phenomena of aging and the problems of older adults, including health, housing, ageism, intergenerational relationships, etc. The particular focus of "public health & aging" on health aspects (conceptualized broadly) related to the aging process sets it as a subfield under gerontology. Throughout this White Paper, then, public health & aging refers to education, training, research, and practice that is oriented to maintaining health and preventing disease among older adults the organizational, community, and societal levels.

Applying public health principles to public health practice with older populations requires knowledge and skills in public health & aging. There needs to be a deliberate transmission of the increasing knowledge of public health and aging to future public health practitioners. This chapter will next examine the demographics of the aging population to show the increasing need for training of new and existing practitioners in public health and aging. It then provides a brief history of the development of training in public health & aging, along with data that describes the current scope and status of professional education in public health & aging. Finally, it offers suggestions about how training might better be structured to improve the applicability of the knowledge, skills, and attitudes which future public health practitioners will need to work with programs and policies that affect older adults.

Demography, Disease, and the Need for Education and Training in Public Health and Aging

The age composition and disease patterns of the country have changed dramatically from that of the past century. At the turn of the 20th century, 40% of the U.S. population was under age 18 while only 4% was age 65 or older.[8] Since the early 20th century there has been a shift in the leading causes of death from infectious (e.g., pneumonia/influenza, tuberculosis) to chronic diseases (e.g., heart disease, cancer, stroke).[9] It is now recognized that behavioral risk factors such as smoking, diet, and exercise significantly contribute to these chronic conditions.[10]

There has also been significant growth in the older population since the early 20th century. Public health has taken a leading role in documenting the incidence and prevalence of chronic conditions and disability in the population, identifying risk factors associated with these problems as well as designing strategies to reduce the risk of chronic diseases, disability, and institutionalization. The continued increase in the numbers of the oldest old will place unrelenting pressure on the health care system, requiring a well educated workforce that includes public health professionals who are prepared to work on health and aging issues.

Origins and Growth of Public Health and Aging

The field of public health and aging is quite recent. While professional research and practice in general public health fostered the founding of the American Public Health Association (APHA) in 1872, the Gerontological Society of America (the primary scientific organization for researchers and educators in gerontology) was not founded until 1945. By 1964 there were still only two schools of public health with courses in public health & aging.[11] Growth in the field led to the formation of a Gerontological Health section in the APHA in 1982, and section membership grew to 1000 in the following ten years. Concern with improving education in the field contributed to the formation of a permanent Task Force on Health & Aging under the auspices of the Association of Schools of Public Health in 1985. By 1992, 21 of 23 accredited U.S. Schools of Public Health surveyed had one or more courses in gerontological public health.[13]

The rapid growth in public health & aging research and training over 10 years was the result of a number of contributing forces: the demographic shift of the population; the development and growth of federal and foundation sponsored research in aging; the recognition of geriatrics as an area of residency training; and the recognition of the need for health professionals who can address issues of long-term care, community based health education interventions and epidemiological health risk factors in older populations.

Politics and Public Health

Through the first half of the 20th century, the primary political involvement of and for older adults involved pensions.[14] Social movements of the aged during the depression focussed on economic issues, centering around publicly funded universal pensions. For a variety of political and economic reasons, Social Security and Old Age Assistance (state administered welfare for the aged) were established at that time.[15] As pensions became a less critical issue, health care for older adults rose in prominence. Although work-based health insurance became common in the U.S. during the 1940s and 1950s, older adults generally were excluded because of their high medical expenses and separation from the labor force.[16] Advocates of national health insurance, having been defeated for years by the medical profession and other special interest groups, shifted their focus to health insurance problems of the older population as a vehicle for developing support for a national health program.[17] The political legitimacy of elderly persons, their need for health insurance, and the social activism of the early 1960s helped the passage of Medicare and Medicaid and boosted awareness of aging as a public health issue.[18] As a discipline that works on improving the health of populations in part by expanding medical care access (both directly through establishing public health clinics and indirectly by improving insurance coverage), the design and implementation of Medicare and Medicaid have been central issues in public health education and research. But Medicare is acute care insurance, and although Medicaid has become a dominant payor of long-term care for the elderly, the public health needs of older adults have been largely unaddressed.

Medicare spending has increased from $8.9 billion in 1972 to $151 billion in 1993.[19] The rapid growth in Medicare and Medicaid expenditures has created political pressure to reduce the use of hospitals and nursing homes,[20] helping to stimulate interest in the public health community in chronic disease prevention and ways of maximizing the independence of the functionally disabled. In addition, the public concern that has been generated regarding Alzheimer's disease has led to increased public health interest in this incurable condition.[21] The high cost associated with chronic conditions such as Alzheimer's disease and the competition for limited health care dollars has contributed to a search for cost effective community-based public health alternatives to institutionalization.

Growth by Research Funding

The demographics and politics of aging has also shaped the research agenda of the country. Federal involvement in health research began in a substantial way with the founding of the National Institutes of Health in 1943 via the Public Health Service Act of 1943 and 1944.[22] In response to the growing recognition of aging research issues, the National Institute on Aging (NIA) was added to NIH in 1974.[23]

While much of NIA's funding goes for biomedical and clinical research, the behavioral sciences section funds a large amount of research that is consistent with a public health perspective. The NIA has sponsored the Established Populations for Epidemiologic

Studies of the Elderly to provide detailed prospective information about the health status of defined older populations. The NIA has also been instrumental in funding national surveys with older populations including the Longitudinal Study of Aging (1984–1990) and the National Caregiver Study (1982–1988). In addition to funding large, longitudinal, national surveys, the NIA issues requests for investigator initiated proposals. Recent initiatives relevant to public health include falls in older adults and physical frailty in older minorities.

The large national surveys funded in part by the NIA have often been conducted and partially funded by the National Center on Health Statistics (NCHS). During the 1980's the agency's interest in aging increased as it produced research and reports on issues of aging and health including determinants of health, use of community-based and long-term care health care services, and assessment of costs associated with the use of such services.[24] Researchers (and program planners) in public health and aging continue to examine these national data sources to better understand the nature of illness and disability in the older population.[25] Books and articles based on these data sources also help provide the knowledge base used in teaching about health and aging.

While the NIA is a major resource for funding public health research with older populations, it is not the only resource contributing to the proliferation of research in public health and aging. Other major research funding sources include the Health Care Financing Administration (HCFA), Agency for Health Care Policy and Research (AHCPR), the National Center for Health Statistics (in co-operation with the Centers for Disease Control), the Administration on Aging (AoA), and the Social Security Administration. Private foundations which have also been funding aging research since the 1960's include the Retirement Research Foundation, the Robert Wood Johnson Foundation and the American Association of Retired Persons (AARP). Together these groups have provided extensive resources that have nurtured gerontological public health research and broadened the knowledge of the health and well being of older adults.

Research has played an important role in the development of gerontological public health training since almost all Schools of Public Health, and most other Masters of Public Health (MPH) programs, are located in large research-oriented universities. As a result, the growing number of researchers in gerontological public health has provided many faculty dispersed over most schools who have been interested in developing public health courses in their area of research expertise. While research has contributed to the foundation of public health and aging, it has also restricted curricula and training in the field. A large proportion of the public health and aging programs are in major academic research centers where research funding and research priorities drive educational policy. While research is not incompatible with public health practice, the rewards for academic faculty are for research activities and not for the application to improving public health practice per se. The Pew Health Professions Commission notes that this problem is common to all academically situated health professions.[26]

Geriatrics, Gerontology, and the Professionalization of Aging Services

There are several conditions that make it possible for a profession to dominate a service sector. Professional dominance generally involves a claim of unique and specialized knowledge, a level of monopoly control over the market for their expertise, required advanced training, and often some type of certification or licensure.[27] Allopathic medicine, nursing, and social work have all followed the path of professional licensure and state regulation that provides them with protected access to a number of gerontological jobs. General gerontology and public health both have accreditation standards for specialized degrees (the MSG and MPH respectively), but neither discipline has the type of privileged access to jobs in the way the other disciplines do.

Programs in gerontology, especially at the master's level, are a relatively recent development. The Older Americans Act, first passed in 1965 and expanded since then, has created an 'aging network' (or aging enterprise) that requires knowledge of aging policy and services that can be met with a degree in gerontology.[28] But gerontology is still attempting to identify a specialized knowledge that it can claim.

Public health is like gerontology in being an interdisciplinary field. However, it is different in having identified a unique methodological tool (epidemiology) and a characteristic intervention approach (health promotion and disease prevention of populations). Public health claims its specialized body of knowledge as involving (1) a broad focus on health and well being, not just the absence of disease and disability; (2) a focus on the aggregate population rather than clinical one-on-one approach; (3) an emphasis on primary and secondary prevention; and (4) interventions at all levels including the person, the family, the community, health care systems, government, and society. The special contribution of this public health approach to aging was codified in a 1990 training curriculum produced for the Bureau of Health Professions.[29] That curriculum, which was targeted at health department employees, covers:

1. Aging, demography, biology, and epidemiology
2. Psychosocial issues in aging and health
3. Financing of the health care of older adults
4. Continuum of care services for older adults and
5. Health promotion for older adults

Similar to graduates with gerontology degrees, public health graduates face competition from those with less education because many public health jobs do not require an accredited MPH degree. The one job that requires a special, accredited degree is that of nursing home administrator. The specific nature of nursing home administrator accreditation requirements, however, results in those degrees being offered more commonly in non-public-health health administration programs than in schools of public health.[30]

Overall, while the process of professionalization has occurred in many of the occupations that work with older adults, the discipline of gerontology and the field of public health have yet to sufficiently communicate to employers the value of their unique body of knowledge, to develop singular control over the market for their expertise, or to require licensure for the practice of their skills. Advanced training is required to obtain the Masters of Science in Gerontology and Masters of Public Health degrees, but those degrees are not necessary requirements for very many jobs.

Summary of Historical Influences

Demography, disease patterns, politics, research funding, and the professionalization of some aging-related disciplines have all contributed to the development of the field of public health and aging. These factors also contribute to the potential for instability in the growth of training in public health and aging. While the demographic shifts and disease patterns are likely to occur as predicted, politics, research funding, and professional turf battles are unpredictable. For example, if research funding opportunities in aging significantly shift from one that is compatible with a public health perspective to one that is more clinical or basic biomedical, there may be a corresponding shift in interest in curriculum and training in public health & aging.

One important factor does *not* currently exist that would encourage training in public health and aging—a strong demand for public health professionals trained specifically in aging issues. Currently, job opportunities are excellent in geriatrics and somewhat unpredictable in gerontology, while a strong demand continues for most licensed health professionals. The demand is softer for personnel in administration, planning, policy analysis, and service delivery jobs where entry-level education and training requirements are frequently loose and unspecialized.[31]

Curriculum Content and Training in Public Health & Aging

A summary of course offerings in aging in U.S. Schools of Public Health (SPH) are provided in Table 2.1. A total of 96 course offerings with content in public health & aging were reported by Schools of Public Health in 1992, compared to 63 course offerings in 1985,[13] an increase of 52 percent over the seven year period. There is a considerable range between universities in the number of aging-related course offerings in schools of public health (0 to 11), with all but two schools offering at least one course in aging.

Table 2.1 also provides a distribution of public health and aging courses offered in 1992 by content area. These SPH courses in public health and aging were categorized into six general topic areas: introduction or overview of public health and aging; processes of aging, (including biology and nutrition in aging); epidemiology; psychosocial issues of aging; organizational finance and delivery of care; and health education and promotion. The content areas were similar to the curricula content areas used in the Geriatric Training Curriculum for Public Health Professionals.[29] Based on this classification, courses in organizational finance and delivery of care were the most common aging courses offered in schools of public health (34 of 96 courses). Seventeen of the 23 schools of public health surveyed had one or more courses in the finance and delivery of care to older populations. The least common public health and aging course offered focused on health education health promotion of older adults (six courses).[13] A broader survey of both schools of public health and accredited programs (n=43) in 1994, found that only half had one or more courses in health and aging.[12]

While individual courses in health and aging are common, coordinated programs on the subject are less common. A review of program literature provided by 23 Schools of Public Health revealed that two offered a special degree in gerontological public health (Table 2.2). Nine programs reported a public health & aging concentration or track. Of the 22 schools that specifically mentioned continuing education, only two discussed public health and aging as part of this continuing education and only four of the 21 schools that reported offering any certificate programs mentioned a certificate in gerontology.[30] This suggests that for most of the schools with a few courses in gerontological public health there are only a few courses offered by faculty with research or applied interests in aging. It appears that most of the gerontological teaching responsibilities in schools without a formal concentration fall on one or a small number of faculty. Thus, the courses may be limited in scope and vulnerable to retirements, changing research interests, and sabbaticals. The low number of schools of public health reporting continuing education in aging suggest that little effort is made at accommodating the public health practitioner who wishes to keep up with current research and best practices in public health and aging.

It is also useful to examine the content of courses since there are many different ways to teach each course topic. A content analysis of 76 syllabi from 18 of the 20 accredited public health programs reporting course work in public health and aging obtained useable information on 71 courses.[34] The most common topics receiving full class sessions in these courses were: a general overview of health policy and aging (39%); non-institutional care of the older population (38%); and normal psychology and mental health (37%) (Table 2.3). Fewer courses devoted one or more class sessions to special populations such as minorities, women, the poor, or the oldest-old, despite the availability of resources that identify the key public health issues in these areas.[32, 33]

Table 2.3 also shows the relative emphasis placed on a broad understanding of health status in older populations in the courses. General health status of older adults is presented in 28 percent of the courses, while issues associated with mental health (23%), chronic physical diseases (15%) and Alzheimer's disease (13%) are also frequently addressed in public health and aging curricula. Extensive course work was also found in the long-term care of chronic conditions including nursing homes (31%), community-based care (38%), and informal care (35%). Overall, most of the existing course work is aimed at students with limited knowledge or experience in gerontology.[31] This means that most students who receive training in aging and public health are receiving a low level of applying public health concepts to the older adult population. This approach is probably appropriate for most public health programs, although there is a need to maintain centers of advanced training where students can take multiple courses that build upon each other so that a continuing stream of students obtain specialized research and practice knowledge and skills that are specific to older adults.

In addition to course content, the way in which courses are taught is important. One major deficiency in public health training, according to the Institute of Medicine's (IOM) report on the Future of Public Health[35] and more recent reports,[3, 4] is a lack of sufficient interaction with agencies and programs addressing the health and social needs of individuals in the community. This failure is also common to courses on health and aging where only one-quarter of the courses reviewed required any first hand experience (e.g. site visit, interview, etc.) with older adults or an organization that works with them.[34] While this type of assignment can be relatively easy to structure, the low incidence of such assignments reflects a broader problem in academic public health of a distancing from the communities and populations served.

The surveys just reviewed[13, 34] from the early 1990s document the growth in public health and aging curricula since the early

1980s. While there is considerable variability in content, curricula are compatible with public health in that they are generally focused on populations rather than individuals and tends to broadly define health in the aggregate population. But the growth in public health and aging is not uniform across either schools of public health or other accredited public health programs. Eight of 23 schools of public health surveyed in 1992 had two or fewer aging courses.[13] In addition, 6 of the 22 accredited MPH programs outside of schools of public health did not report any formal course content in aging.[34] In addition, there is little movement to develop credentialing or specific degrees in aging and public health at this time.

Analyses of gerontological public health curricula reflect forces that have encouraged the development of the field. The demographic and disease patterns of older adults generated from research using national data are well reflected in public health curricula. The considerable research in long-term care services and political and public concern over funding health services for the older population is reflected in the large proportion of public health and aging courses in organization, finance and delivery of care. The politics of aging has helped produce more course content on Alzheimer's disease than on death and dying, but overall the focus of courses is even more likely to reflect central public health concerns such as successful or "healthy" aging and health promotion through modified health behavior. Finally, the limited professionalization in public health (not to mention gerontological public health) has resulted in a plethora of introductory aging courses in public health training programs and few advanced courses and little exposure to field experience and public health practice in aging.

Future Directions for Training in Public Health and Aging

Some forces that shape existing training in public health & aging are likely to continue into the future. Demographic and disease patterns of the population will continue to create a need for professionals with knowledge and skills relevant to the aged. In addition, the growing numbers and high medical care consumption by older adults will continue to generate political pressure for both continued research in health problems faced by older adults, as well as continued attempts at cost containment. The evolving health care system is likely to lead some disciplines such as social work and nursing to further expand their roles in some health and aging services (e.g., case management within managed care).

Cost containment efforts are stimulating growth in areas that need more personnel trained in public health and aging. In particular, providing medical care in managed care systems has become a favored method of controlling costs. A small proportion of older persons are currently in managed care, but the number will grow rapidly in coming years. Older persons pose different problems than younger adults for managed care, making knowledge in public health and aging important for health administrators and policy makers in this arena. Cost containment in the public sector is also targeting other provider reimbursement issues, long term care, retiree health benefits, and other topics. The development and implementation of these policies in ways that protects and promotes the health of older persons requires a broad dissemination of knowledge in health and aging to health care policy makers and administrators.

Health promotion and disease prevention targeted at populations or groups of older

Table 2.1 Number and Distribution of Public Health & Aging Courses by School of Public Health and Courses Content Area 1992

School of Public Health	A	B	C	D	E	F	Total	1985
University of Alabama-Birmingham					1	1	2	0
Boston University	1		1		2		4	2
University of California-Berkeley		1		1	3	1	6	3
University of California-Los Angeles	1		1	3	3	1	9	2
Columbia University	1	3		2	5		11	8
Harvard University							0	1
University of Hawaii	2	1		1	1		5	6
University of Illinois-Chicago	1	1	1	2	3	1	9	4
Johns Hopkins University	1	1	1		1	1	5	4
Loma Linda University	2	1	1	1			5	3
University of Massachusetts					1		1	0
University of Michigan		2	1	2	1		6	8
University of Minnesota	2	2			2		6	4
University of North Carolina	1	1		1	4		7	4
University of Oklahoma			1	1	1	1	3	4
University of Pittsburgh			2	1	1		4	2
San Diego State University							0	0
University of South Carolina		2	1		1		4	0
University of South Florida		1					1	0
University of Texas					1		1	2
Tulane University	1				3		4	0
University of Washington							1	1
Yale University	1		1				2	5
Totals	**14**	**16**	**11**	**15**	**34**	**6**	**96**	**63**

A. Introduction/overview of aging; D. Psycho-social issues of Aging; B. Processes of Aging; E. Organizational finance/delivery of care; C. Epidemiology of Aging; F. Health education/health promotion in aging

Table 2.2 Percent of Content Areas Covered in One or More Public Health & Aging Class Sessions (n=71)

HEALTH PROBLEMS & HEALTH SERVICES	
Health status, general	28%
Mental health, psychology	35%
Mental illness	23%
Alzheimer's & dementias	13%
Chronic disease	15%
Dying	7%
Health care organization, general	11%
Acute care	6%
Nursing home	31%
Alternative (community) services	38%
Informal care/family	35%
DISEASE PREVENTION & HEALTH PROMOTION	
Health promotion/prevention	24%
Teaching methods	4%
Normal/successful aging	21%
Autonomy & independence	7%
Health behavior	24%
Social construction of aging or health	21%
Social issues (e.g. retirement)	17%
PRACTICE ISSUES	
Program planning	11%
Program evaluation/assessment	10%
Administration/management	11%
Quality assurance/quality of care	23%
Ethics	20%
SPECIAL POPULATIONS	
Minority aged	20%
Older women	8%
Socio-economic status (SES)	10%
Oldest old (85+)	3%
POLICY ISSUES	
Health policy - overview	39%
Regulation	15%
Finance, general	23%
Cost-containment	8%
Medicaid/Medicare	8%
Private insurance	8%
Policy process	14%
Political power - elderly organizations	11%
OTHER ISSUES	
Demography of aging	28%
Epidemiology	21%
Biology of aging	25%
Gerontological & related theory	20%
Research methods in aging	15%
International issues	1%

adults, on the other hand, are unlikely to increase as a result of evolutionary changes in the health care system. The nature of these programs results in long-term rather than short term fiscal savings and improvements in the quality of life that are difficult to quantify. While individual hospitals and insurance companies can be capitated to provide medical services, the "public" nature of public health necessitates a governmental role. This governmental role includes active support of higher education in public health and aging to produce a future workforce with the appropriate knowledge and skills for an aging society.

The growth of the aging population and its complicated health and disease issues will continue to generate a demand for health professionals with *some* knowledge of public health & aging. The small number of students who take graduate coursework in health and aging nationally indicates that few students obtain this knowledge through specialized coursework. Current accreditation standards require that public health professional students receive training in five core areas of public health: epidemiology, biostatistics, behavioral sciences, environmental health, and health services. While each of these areas are important to older adults, there is no guarantee that students will receive any training in how to apply those subject areas to policies and programs for older adults. It is important that the older population be referenced throughout the core curriculum so that *all* students develop an awareness of older adults as a significant target of all public health measures, and not simply a group that is only of concern to hospital and nursing home administrators.

A workshop on public health and aging[36] identified six areas where public health professional students should ideally be able to demonstrate competence:

1. A basic understanding of biological, psychological, social, and environmental aspects of health and illness in the aging process
2. An understanding of the changing aging population and its interaction with society and the health care system
3. An appreciation of the heterogeneity of the older adult population and the aging process
4. The ability to integrate public health & aging research into practice
5. Skills and knowledge in the organization and delivery of services to older adults
6. A sensitivity to moral, ethical and legal issues in aging

In addition to the need for all public health professionals to have a general sensitivity to aging issues, there will be a continuing need for public health practitioners who have specialized in health and aging. These professionals will staff the front-line in program planning, implementation, management, and direct service delivery. While those professionals need the six competencies listed above, they require more in-depth training in the complex issues that face older adults. The health and aging workshop noted earlier[36] identified the following 15 subject areas that should be included in a curriculum for students specializing in health and aging:

1. Theories of Aging and Normal Aging (including basic biology of aging)
2. Epidemiology
3. Aging and a healthy environment
4. Health promotion in aging populations
5. The older adult and the acute care system
6. Chronic illness
7. Organization, financing, and delivery of long-term care
8. Mental health and mental illness
9. Informal support and family systems
10. Death and dying
11. Organizational cultures and health care
12. Diversity issues (race, ethnicity, gender)
13. Politics of Aging
14. Issues in research, program design, and education of older adults
15. Ethics of health and aging

While these subjects could be covered in a single course, further training in some of the topics is desirable.

Future growth in the training of public health and aging professionals must also address the needs of practitioners in the

Table 2.3 Public Health & Aging Program Characteristics for Schools of Public Health, 1992

School of Public Health	Degree Programs	Track, or con-concentration specialization	Continuing Education	Certificate Programs
University of Alabama-Birmingham	No	No	No	No
Boston University	No	Yes	No	No
University of California-Berkeley	No	No	No	No
University of CA-Los Angeles	No	Yes	No	No
Columbia University	Yes	Yes	Yes	No
Harvard University	No	No	No	No
University of Hawaii	No	No	No	No
University of Illinois-Chicago	No	Yes	Yes	Yes
Johns Hopkins University	Yes	*	*	Yes
Loma Linda University	No	Yes	*	*
University of Massachusetts	No**	No	*	*
University of Michigan	No	No	No	No
University of Minnesota	No	Yes	No	No
University of North Carolina	No	No	No	No
University of Oklahoma	No	No	No	No
University of Pittsburgh	No	Yes	No	No
San Diego State University	No	No	No	No
University of South Carolina	No	No	*	Yes
University of South Florida	No***	Yes	No	Yes
University of Texas	No	No	No	No
Tulane University	No	No	No	No
University of Washington	No	No	No	No
Yale University	No	No	No	No
TOTALS	**2**	**9**	**2**	**4**

* Unable to determine from materials

** Ph.D. in Gerontology (Graduate School, not school of public health)

*** M.A. in Gerontology (College of Arts and Sciences, not school of public health)

community. Because a significant proportion of the public health workforce does not have a strong public health background, it is also important that continuing education be available and encouraged for those already in the workforce. Perhaps most surprising in the review of aging courses in Schools of Public Health was the limited availability of continuing education training in the area.[13] The absence of licensure requirements guarantees that people from a variety of backgrounds will be in positions that involve public health and aging. This can be good when it brings a variety of perspectives and experiences that are useful in problem solving and program development. But, it is a problem when the diversity of training brings uneven levels of knowledge about the issues facing the aged, limited knowledge about what has worked and not worked in the past, and/or a lack of appreciation of how generic programs and policies need to be modified to best address older individuals. In the aging network (primarily Area Agencies on Aging), employees report a high level of need in job relevant continuing education, including information on aging policies and regulations, data on community resources and funding, and knowledge about alternative ways of meeting the needs of older adults.[37] These are areas that would also be relevant to public health professionals who work in the aging field.

The challenges of developing and evaluating successful public health policies and interventions for older adults will require a cadre of well-trained public health academic researchers. These academics are also needed to teaching graduate-level health and aging courses. To adequately train such academics will require the maintenance of several accredited public health programs which have well-developed concentrations in health and aging. While it appears that the current number of such programs is adequate, those centers of excellence in research need to continue to receive continuing support so that this type of training remains an institutional priority in those universities.

Conclusions

Accredited programs in public health promote the advancement of public health by producing graduates educated and skilled in the field of public health, conducting research, serving as primary resources to government and other entities at all levels, collaborating with other schools and departments within the university, and providing education and training for current practitioners. These same service and educational objectives should be followed for public health students in aging. A number accredited programs educate students in public health for work in agencies which deliver services to older adults in the community. This is particularly true of Masters of Public Health (MPH) and Doctor of Public Health (DrPH) degrees which are directed toward public health students interested in service and administrative positions.

A fundamental shortcoming of academic education and training of public health and aging professionals is that it often fails to adequately communicate with the community agencies providing health and social services for older adults. The Public Health Faculty/Agency Forum addressed this lack of adequate links between public health schools and public health agencies.[3] They recommended the development of formal programs between schools and agencies, thereby creating permanent practicum slots in which students would regularly rotate through an agency. To better link academic faculty and community practitioners they suggested faculty taking part-time appointments at community agencies, agency staff gaining appointments in Schools of Public Health, and temporary faculty/agency exchanges. A reciprocal exchange of information and expertise would benefit students, professionals in community agencies serving older populations, and ultimately, older community residents.

If public health expects to be effective in responding to the needs of older adults in the community, public health educators need to work with programs and community groups typically not pursued by academic institutions. Educational institutions that prepare the public health workforce need to respond to the growing importance of community-based organizations that are becoming increasingly central in meeting the demands for community care of older persons. As the Institute of Medicine notes,[35] to achieve public health objectives, public health will need to serve as leaders and catalyst of private efforts as well as performing those health functions that only government can perform.

The increase in research and information on aging and public health has resulted in the development of curriculum resource materials tailored to specific health care disciplines within public health (e.g.[29, 38]). However, at this time every accredited program in public health does not need to have a full degree, track, concentration, or specialization in public health and aging. Given the demographic and historical influences discussed earlier, all programs should offer at least one elective and include material on the older adults as examples of how to implement programs and policies relating to each of the core areas in required core courses. It may not be possible to guarantee that everyone working in gerontological public health has specialized in the field, but all public health professionals should be are aware of the issues of this growing population.

Despite the growing need public health professionals who are trained in health and aging, accredited MPH programs nationally reported that only 5% of their students enrolled in a class on health and aging in 1993.[12] At least two changes could make training in health and aging more responsive to the labor market. First, public health organizations and agencies could emphasize perspectives compatible primarily with the field of public health and aging (e.g., community based health promotion and disability prevention for older populations). A beginning of this exists in the form of a small chronic disease prevention block grant that the federal government provides states. The demand for those trained in public health and aging is unlikely to catch the attention of educators and students, however, until funding reaches the magnitude of smoking control or AIDS prevention. The second labor market change that would encourage training in aging and public health would be for jobs in working with older adults to give a clear preference to those with gerontological training. Establishing job preferences, however, generally assumes an adequate supply of appropriately trained professionals in the workforce. Building this critical capacity can be facilitated by providing priority funding for workforce education in public health and aging. These changes are likely to lead public health educators to shape curricula to more directly meet the needs of potential employers in the field of health and aging, thereby improving the quality and effectiveness of public health programs that affect aging Americans.

RECOMMENDATIONS

Educational Issues

1. Increase linkages between public health and aging networks through education, training, and collaboration

Rationale

The need for interaction between public health and aging networks has become increasingly evident as the population has aged and demographic and health imperatives have blurred some of the distinctions between the two fields. In general, public health and aging have had differing histories, philosophies, policies, and funding streams. Public health has the longer history focusing on community-wide solutions to infectious disease and environmental issues. More recently, health promotion and disease prevention have become targets of public health for the Year 2000. The development of the aging network was initiated in this century and focused on services that would maintain the independence of older adults within the community and delay their institutionalization. Until recently, the fields have functioned relatively independently of one another, even while their concerns and target populations were beginning to merge. In order to stimulate closer working relationships between public health and aging agencies, mechanisms that facilitate those relationships and enhance education, training and collaboration between the two groups need to be initiated. Schools of Public Health are in a unique position to influence the development of collaboration between these agencies. To keep pace with increases in the older population by the turn of the century, there would have to be a corresponding increase in public health professionals who receive education and training in aging and public health.

Actions Required

1) Develop innovative projects in curriculum design directed towards improving the health of older adults by increasing the linkages between public health and aging networks in order to facilitate:

- the development of practitioner/faculty team taught courses in public health and aging reflecting the perspective of agencies who service older populations and the academic community;
- the involvement of representatives from health departments and the area agencies on aging (AAA) in the design of courses;
- the development of student internships in public health and aging agencies;
- the inclusion of representatives from public health and aging agencies on the boards of directors of each other's agency; and,
- the employment of graduates of these programs in both agencies;

2) Provide a grant mechanism to accredited programs in public health to facilitate the design and evaluation of these projects. 3. Collaborate with state health departments to develop strategic plans for aged populations.

Responsible Agents

1) State and local departments of aging; 1–3. state and local departments of public health; 1. BHPr Education;
2) Administration of Aging in collaboration with the Bureau of Health Professions.

Expected Outcomes

1a) Over a five-year period there will be a minimum of a 20% increase in:

- the numbers of courses and students in public health and aging programs;
- representatives from health departments and aging agencies serving on curriculum committees in schools of public health; and
- courses with participation by public health and aging practitioners.

1b) There will also be increases in the numbers of health professional students who have had internships in each of these

agencies by one a year; 1c. increases in the numbers of professionals from public health and aging agencies who serve on each others' board of directors or key committees by two a year; 1d. increases in the number of students from accredited public health and aging programs who are employed by public health and aging agencies by two a year.
2) Within three years, at least five grants will be awarded to accredited schools of public health to design and evaluate these innovative projects.
3) Within five years there will be a 20% increase in the numbers of state health departments that have developed strategic plans for the aging population.

2. Expand continuing education in public health and aging; Improve opportunities for life-long learning

Rationale

Information pertaining to the public health of older adults is increasing rapidly resulting in the need for continued training of public health and aging by public health practitioners. While the public health profession has become increasingly aware of the health needs of the older population, the majority of public health professionals working with the older population have little or no formal training in the area of public health and aging. Presently there are only two continuing education programs in public health and aging. Because of this shortage of public health practitioners trained in aging and the continued need to educate current public health professionals on advances in public health issues, the need for continuing education in public health and aging should assume a priority. Academic institutions and programs in public health and aging are resources to meet the need for continuing education to both public health professionals and state/regional policy makers.

Actions Required

1) Development, implementation, and evaluation of regionally available ongoing continuing education programs which provide public health practitioners with research and current best practices in aging;
2) Development of model continuing education programs which educate policy makers at the state and regional level on issues pertaining to public health and aging;
3) Collaboration between academic institutions in public health and aging and public health agencies to tailor and expand continuing education offerings to provide career development tracks for professionals interested in public health and aging.

Responsible Agents

1) Geriatric Education Centers; 1–3. Academic Programs in Public Health and Aging;
2) Bureau of Health Professions, Foundations; State and local legislative bodies; 1–3. State health agencies with practitioners in public health and aging.

Expected Outcomes

1) Within five years 50% of the continuing education programs in public health and aging will be based on a model of continuing education with state public health agencies;
2) Over five years new educational programs will be offered at three major conferences of public officials. The new conference programs will attract officials and/or staff from at least 40 different states (or 50% of the appropriate geographic unit) over the period of three years;
3) Within five years there will be an

increase of 50% in continuing education programs that are oriented to career development in public health and aging.

3. Develop methods and standards for timely information dissemination of advances in public health and aging to practitioners in aging and the general public

Rationale

The 1988 Institute of Medicine report has called attention to the dual responsibility of Public Health Schools in conducting research and educating public health practitioners. The 1990 Pew report on The Future of Public health Professions has stressed the need for schools of public health to interface with the public health profession. They note that schools of public health can function as a means of rapid transfer of intellectual and/or technological advances achieved within the university to the health care needs of the public. In order for this to be accomplished, academic programs in public health must develop methods to promote the timely transfer and dissemination of research advances in public health and aging into understandable and practical information for the public and public health professions. They must also develop skills in public health professionals on methods of information dissemination in public health and aging.

Actions Required

1) Development of Public Health and Aging curricula and training materials for academic professionals in public health and aging on how to apply and disseminate current research and best practices in aging for consumption by the general public, public health practitioners and public health agencies;

2) Development of continuing education to assist public health professionals to interpret and apply current research and best practices in aging.

Responsible Agents

1–2. Public Health Schools and Programs, Bureau of Health Professions, Health Agencies, Foundations, Public Health Agencies, Aging Agencies, Association of Academic Health Centers.

Expected Outcomes

Within five years 50% of accredited Public Health and Aging programs will:

1) Design and implement one or more courses on how to apply and disseminate current research and best practices in aging for consumption by the general public, public health practitioners and public health agencies;

2) Provide training for public health and aging practitioners on how to translate and apply current research and best practices into action.

4. Implement new technologies which facilitate learning and communication between aging programs in schools of public health and public health practitioners in aging.

Rationale

Even with an additional emphasis on training and continuing education in public health and aging, a shortage of professionals in public health and aging will remain for the near future. Without technology which facilitates education and training beyond the walls of academic institutions, the task of meeting the needs of public health professionals to be adequately trained in aging will fall short. Technologies that promote interactive learning and multiply the opportunity for education in public health and aging are needed to help meet these shortages. Technologies such as interactive video-teleconferencing and video related products are also needed to facilitate distance learning and bring advances in public health and aging to health practitioners in remote sites. The need for these new communication and education technologies are great for public health practitioners in aging as well as students in programs in public health and aging.

Actions Required

1) Creation of demonstration programs which introduce and evaluate new technologies designed to facilitate communication, educational opportunities and exchange of information between academic institutions in public health and aging and agencies serving older adults;
2) Implementation of innovative technologies with demonstrated value in facilitating communication and exchange of information between public health and aging programs and agencies serving older adults.

Responsible Agents

1–2. Schools and Programs in Public Health, Bureau of Health Professions in concert with Foundations.

Expected Outcomes

1) Within one year, at least two schools of public health will be funded to develop, pilot and evaluate innovative technologies designed to facilitate communication and learning between schools of public health and public health and aging practitioners;
2) Within five years, a model program to apply innovative educational technologies and interactive learning for public health and aging will be made available for use in programs.

Attitudes and Perceptions of the Older Adult Population

5. Improve the knowledge and attitudes of public health students about older persons

Rationale

Most public health students do not consider the older person as a priority target for public health interventions. Students have little knowledge about the potentials for health promotion, disease prevention, and health policy that are of substantial benefit to older persons. Public health grew out of an emphasis on sanitary reform and maternal-child health issues, and has failed to fully adapt to the changing health challenges of the nation. Since most public health practitioners will have an impact on the health of the older adults, all students need a minimum knowledge of health and aging issues and some students should have substantial knowledge. Universities currently provide training in health and aging in a variety of ways, without the benefit of any consensus on the most effective means of organizing public health and aging education. Training in health and aging can be improved by determining the appropriateness and effectiveness of different educational strategies.

Actions Required

1) Encourage core public health courses to include health and aging materials by developing new materials and model standards, and offering small grants to implement them; 2. Fund research to determine the relative impact of different curricular strategies for training effective specialists in public health and aging; 3. Require public health accreditation self-studies to explain how health and aging is represented in their curricula or justify its absence.

Responsible Agents

1–2) Bureau of Health Professions; 1–2. Foundations; 1–3. Accredited Programs in Public Health; 3. Council on Education in Public Health.

Expected Outcomes

1) Increase by 50% the number of social/behavioral science core courses with content on health and aging in accredited public health programs;
2) Information on the most effective strategies of training will lead 10% of nonconforming programs to change the program structure within three years after the report;
3) Accreditation self-studies will all discuss the role of health and aging in pubic health.

6. Increase the attention of public health education and practice to issues of diversity among older adults

Rationale

Diversity among the older adults is created by those with health, cultural, and/or social characteristics that make "standard" health programs less effective. Examples include:
1) Racial and ethnic minorities whose culture and social status must be addressed in health promotion and disease treatment;
2) Rural residence where geographic dispersion is a barrier to health care. To maximize efficiency and effectiveness we must tailor programs and services to the target populations. Public health is distinguished by focus on populations and groups, making it a lead discipline in identifying and educating primary care professionals in the social and cultural aspects of health and healing. But even in public health there is limited attention given to diversity among the older adults; only 20% of public health courses include one or more class session on racial and ethnic minorities, 8% on older women, and 3% on the oldest old (age 85+). Rural aging is a largely neglected topic.

Actions Required

1) Increase faculty awareness through disseminating materials on diversity, expanding faculty development opportunities, and offering consultation in curriculum development on the topic;
2) Increase course content on diversity by improving the curricular materials available; including the production of new and innovative course materials, improving dissemination, and establishing core competencies in ethnogerontology and public health;
3) Increase the number of public health students in field training sites that have programs for diverse populations, through developing faculty internships and BHPr Special Projects funding for student internship development;
4) Increase the diversity of the students taking public health and aging course by offering stipends, attractive internships, and links with diverse communities.

Responsible Agents

1–4. Bureau of Health Professions; 1–4. other professional organizations; 1–4. Foundations; Accredited Public Health Programs; 1–2. Association of Schools of Public Health; 3–4. Administration on Aging.

Expected Outcomes

1) Disseminate new curricular materials to all accredited public health programs and establish a mechanism for improving future dissemination by building on BHPr's Minority Aging curriculum conference/book, the American Association of Retired Persons applied research series, Carnegie's Aging Society Project, and GSA's minority aging workshops;

2a) Increase the number of courses with material on diversity by 20% over five years. Increase the number of public health students in those courses by 15% over five years;
2b) Develop key competencies, disseminate to all accredited public health programs, and incorporate competencies into half of appropriate courses over three years;
3) BHPr Special Projects grants include priorities for aging and underrepresented populations;
4a) Increase the number of MPH students in diversity internships by 15% over three years;
4b) Increase by 20% the number of students from underrepresented minorities who take one or more courses in health and aging over three years.

Strategic Plans and Other Administrative Issues and Evaluation

7. Promote interdisciplinary practice through interdisciplinary role socialization in accredited public health programs.

Rationale

The provision of seamless and coordinated health programs for aging populations demands collaborative practice and programmatic skills contributed by interdisciplinary teams. Academic health professions education today remains challenged to create curriculum processes which can blend the core skills of professionals in a manner that preserves the unique knowledge and skill required for interdisciplinary effectiveness. Hallmark reports by PEW and others in the 1990s are challenging traditional, disciplinary philosophies of preparation by calling for health practitioners who understand and value interdisciplinary efforts. The knowledge, attitudes and skills required to provide interdisciplinary practice are absent in current academic structures and curriculum. Interdisciplinary role models among teaching faculty and clinicians have remained invisible and undervalued except through federal and foundation funded programs.

Actions Required

1) Institute and evaluate prescribed theoretical and clinical coursework in collaboration, critical thinking and conflict management. Require for all levels of health professions students interdisciplinary practicum experiences in which interdisciplinary teams are evaluated on the efficiency and effectiveness of their teaming efforts to resolve critical community problems with aged populations;
2) Institute enabling language in federal and state health professions education legislation and set funding preference and priority initiatives for interdisciplinary education in public health and aging.

Responsible Agents

1) Accrediting bodies for Schools and Programs of Public Health; 1–2. Foundation initiated ventures; BHPr sponsored faculty development initiatives; professional organization position papers.

Expected Outcomes

1) At least 50% of public health programs require theoretical and practical interdisciplinary coursework and project activities within 5 years;
1–2) Interdisciplinary courses will evaluate pretest—post test changes in attitudes toward a collaborative mode of professional behaviors as measured on standardized tests (such as, Thomas Kilmann); responses to post-graduation surveys report the use of collaborative skills in practice at 1, 3 and 5 years.

8. Stabilize public health education funding

Rationale

Unlike the entitlement mechanism currently funding Graduate Medical Education, health professions funding at the federal level is subject to discretionary, renewable and unstable funding streams. Entitlement education funding for public health professionals is now warranted to tie the funding levels of public health professionals to distribution of providers and health status indicators congruent with the *Healthy People 2000* objectives. Health professions funding must reinforce primary health care skills and curriculums capable of producing graduates with the core public health functions for aging adults. In the future older adults will utilize a larger share of public health resources and organized services for safe environments, chronic disease prevention and control, and effective health behaviors.

Actions Required

1) Institute a National Strategic Planning Process to link health professions production for 2005 with *Healthy People 2000 Objectives*;
2) Change funding mechanism at federal and state levels from discretionary to entitlement procedures in fiscal planning;
3) Develop federal and state initiatives for programmatic, faculty development and student support in public health/aging through health professions funding initiatives;
4) Develop cooperative health professions funding initiatives for joint program implementation in public health and aging between schools of public health, nursing, and other health professions schools.

Responsible Agents

1) U.S. Department of Health and Human Services, Public Health Service, Bureau of Health Professions; 1., 3., 4. PEW Foundation; 1–2. National Association of Governors; and 1–2., 4. Professional Education Organizations; 3–4. Department of Labor and Education; 1–2. American Association for Retired Persons.

Expected Outcomes

1, 3, 4) National Strategic Plan published in three years reflects workforce strategies, resources, and health status indicators sensitive to older adults;
1–2) National Governors Association endorses plan and implements resources for appropriate workforce development, funding and distribution within 3–5 years in the states;
1–4). Health professions shortage areas (HPSA) are reduced by 50% by 2000;
4) Numbers of students graduating with masters and doctoral degrees will increase by 150 during first five years;
1–2) The number of public health professionals educated in geriatrics and public health is increased by 50% by 2000.

9. Establish standardized credentialing options for institutions to insure minimum and continued competencies in public health and aging

Rationale

The Institute of Medicine (1988) analysis of public health and public health education during the last two decades reveals the difficulties presented by a lack of clear mission and consistent educational arrangements. Public health practitioners may have graduated from an accredited school of public health, a health education program, a community medicine program, a school of nursing or one of the 69 non accredited programs offering the MPH/MSPH degree. In addition, over 300 programs offer public-health-related degrees in non accredited programs (PEW, 1993). Standardized credentialing for programs preparing public health/aging professionals is absent. Likewise, credentialing mechanisms for continued competency and professional development would contribute to a responsible oversight structure and process for public health practitioners. Similarly, gerontology professionals are typically prepared in programs absent of curriculum content and experiences in public health. Standardized credentialing programs are one mechanism to offer post graduate educational offerings for practicing public health and aging professionals. This mechanism is especially important where barriers to additional degrees exit.

Actions Required

1) Analyze type, number and impact of current credentialing resources for public health and gerontology providers;
2) Analyze existing skill levels of practitioners through a contract for task analysis at the federal level;
3) Fund and evaluate demonstration projects to identify and measure competencies for public health and aging providers;
4) Develop and publish a model scope, standards of practice and competency credentialing program that can be implemented by 1998; 5. Institute the requirement for content in lifespan development in order to receive programmatic accreditation for public health and aging.

Responsible Agents

1–2, 4) American Public Health Association;
1–4) Public Health Service - BHPr;
1, 4, 5) Association of Schools of Public Health;
1, 3) Foundations;
2, 4) American Nurses Credentialing Center.

Expected Outcomes

1–4) A report on status of professional competency mechanisms and impact is published in three years;
1–5) Task analysis provides a foundation for competency measures, credentialing models, and curriculum development;
3–4) Two demonstration projects on credentialing are funded with outcomes disseminated in five years;
4–5) Model scope of practice, standards of practice and competency credentialing program published in three years.

10. Evaluate the implementation of these goals

Rationale

Many of the recommendations presented here require data that does not currently exist to establish baseline patterns and trends. To determine the progress being made towards the goals, and the effectiveness and efficiency of these initiatives, requires ongoing monitoring of public health education.

Actions Required

1) Conduct biannual survey of courses, curriculum, faculty, students, and programs to establish baseline levels and assess implementation of goals;
2) Disseminate findings and information on most successful programs.

Responsible Agents

1–2) Bureau of Health Professions;
1–2) Foundations.

Expected Outcomes

1) Develop a longitudinal database on public health and aging curriculum, faculty, and students;
2) Publish and publicize biannually a report on the implementation of these recommen-

dations, and identify the barriers to the achievement of any unrealized goals.

REFERENCES

1. U.S. Public Health Service. Healthy people 2000 : National health promotion and disease prevention objectives. Washington, DC: U.S. Department of Health and Human Services. 1991.
2. AARP. Healthy People 2000: Healthy Older Adults. Washington, DC: American Association of Retired Persons. 1991.
3. Sorensen AA, Bialek RG. The Public Health Faculty/Agency Forum Final Report: Linking Graduate Education and Practice. Gainesville, Florida: University Press of Florida. 1991.
4. Pew Health Professions Commission. Primary Care Workforce 2000: Federal Policy Paper. San Francisco, CA: Center for the Health Professions. 1994.
5. Ibrahim MA, Osborn JE. "Future of the Public Health Profession." Pp. 35–44 in E.H. O'Neil and D.M. Hare, eds., Perspectives on the Health Professions. Durham, NC: PEW Health Professions Programs, Duke University. 1990.
6. Larson PF, Osterweis M, Rubin ER. Health workforce issues for the 21st century. Washington, DC: Association of Academic Health Centers. 1994.
7. Denton DR. Caring for An Aging Society: Issues and Strategies for Gerontology Education. Atlanta, GA: SREB. 1990.
8. U.S. Senate, Special Committee on Aging. Aging America, Trends and Projections. Washington, DC: U.S. DHHS. 1991.
9. McKinlay JB, McKinlay SM, Beaglehold R. Trends in death and disease and the contribution of medical measures. Pp. 14–45 in Freeman HE, Levine S, Handbook of Medical Sociology. 4th ed. Englewood Cliffs, NJ: Prentice Hall, 1989.
10 Institute of Medicine. The second 50 years: Promoting health and preventing disability. Washington, DC: National Academy Press, 1992.
11. Magee J., Gerontology Programs and Curricula in U.S. Schools of Public Health. Bureau of Health Professions, U.S. PHS, DHHS. 84–213. Washington, DC: Association of Schools of Public Health. 1985.
12. Wallace SP, Lubben J. Status of Gerontological Training in Public Health and Social Work Programs. Los Angeles, CA: UCLA/California Geriatric Education Center, 1995.
13. Prohaska T. The current status of training in aging and public health. In Wallace SP, Prohaska T, Proceedings from the Aging and Public Health Curriculum Development Workshop. Los Angeles, CA: California Geriatric Education Center, UCLA, 1992.
14. Wallace SP, Williamson JB, Lung RG, Powell LA. "A Lamb in Wolf's Clothing? The Reality of Senior Power and Social Policy." Pp. 95–114 In M. Minkler and C.L. Estes, Critical Perspectives on Aging. Amityville, NY: Baywood, 1991.
15. Quadagno J. The Transformation of Old Age Security. Berkeley, CA: University of California Press, 1988.
16. Fein R., Medical Care, Medical Costs. Cambridge, MA: Harvard. 1989.
17. Starr P., The Social Transformation of American Medicine. New York: Basic Books. 1982.
18. Wallace, SP, Williamson JB. "The Senior Movement in Historical Perspective." In Wallace SP and Williamson JB, The Senior Movement. New York: G.K. Hall. 1992.
19. Levit KR, Sensenig AL, Cowan CA, Lazenby HC, McDonnell PA, Won DK, et al. National health expenditures, 1993. Health Care Financing Review. 16(1):247–294, 1994.
20. Estes CL, Swan JH, and Associates. The Long-term Care Crisis: Elders Trapped in the No-Care Zone. Newbury Park, CA: Sage. 1993.
21. Fox P. "From Senility to Alzheimer's Disease: The Rise of the Alzheimer's Disease Movement." Milbank Quarterly. 67(1):58–102. 1989.

22. Snyder L. Public Health Service Act, 1944. Public Health Reports, 109, 4, 468–471. 1994.
23 Lockett BA. Aging, Politics, and Research: Setting the Federal Agendas for Research on Aging. New York: Springer. 1983.
24. National Center for Health Statistics. Vital and Health Statistics Health Data on Older Americans, 1992. U.S. Department of Health and Human Services (PHS) Series 3, No. 27. 1993.
25. Harris T, Kovar M. Data sets for research in aging: The National Center for Health Statistics, p.248–261. In R. Wallace and R. Woolson (Eds.) The Epidemiologic Study of the Elderly, Oxford University Press, New York. 1992.
26. Sugars DA, O'Neil EH, Bader JD. Healthy America: Practitioners for 2005, An agenda for action for U.S. health professions schools. Durham, NC: Pew Health Professions Commission. 1991.
27. Larson MS. The Rise of Professionalism. Berkeley, CA: University of California Press. 1977.
28. Estes CL. The Aging Enterprise. San Francisco: Jossey-Bass, 1979.
29. U.S. Bureau of Health Professions. Geriatric Training Curriculum for Public Health Professionals. Washington, DC: Department of Health and Human Services (PHS) Health Resources and Services Administration. 1990.
30. Infeld L, Kress JR. Crisis or Quality: Management for Long-term Care. McLean, VA: Association of University Programs in Health Administration. 1989.
31. Kahl A. Career preparation in public health and aging. In S.P. Wallace and T. Prohaska, eds., Proceedings from the Aging and Public Health Curriculum Development Workshop. Los Angeles, CA: California Geriatric Education Center and UCLA School of Public Health. 1992.
32. Torres-Gil F. Hispanics in an Aging Society. From a conference sponsored by the Aging Society Project of Carnegie Corporation of New York. New York: Carnegie Corp. 1986.
33. Harper MS. Minority Aging: Essential Curricula Content for Selected Health and Allied Health Professions. Washington, DC: Bureau of Health Professions, HRSA, PHS. 1990.
34. Wallace SP. The contribution of public health to gerontology: An evaluation of public health curricula on aging. Gerontology and Geriatrics Education, 14(4), 21–37. 1994.
35. Institute of Medicine. The Future of Public Health, National Academy Press, Washington D.C. 1988.
36. Wallace SP, Prohaska T. Proceedings from the Aging and Public Health Curriculum Development Workshop. Los Angeles, CA: California Geriatric Education Center, UCLA. 1992.
37. Peterson DA, Wendt PF, Douglass EB. Determining the Impact of Gerontology Preparation on Personnel in the Aging Network: A National Survey. Washington, DC: Association for Gerontology in Higher Education. 1991.
38. Haber D. Health Promotion and Aging. New York: Springer. 1994.

3

Social Work

Barbara Berkman, Rose Dobrof, Lois Harry, and Joan Damron-Rodriguez

THE STATE OF THE ART OF GERIATRIC SOCIAL WORK EDUCATION AND TRAINING

Introduction

Foundations of Social Work Practice with Older Adults and Their Families

The demand for social work services in the field of aging will be increasing through the year 2020. Major factors affecting this demand for social workers include the rapidly-increasing numbers of persons 65 years of age and older, particularly the rapidly growing population of older adults at high risk for social, psychological and environmental problems (i.e., the minority aged, women, people over age 75, and those with chronic illnesses). Within the changing health care environment, there will be increased need for social, emotional and environmental support services for the elderly. Concomitantly, there will be even greater need for geriatric social work education.

This chapter will illuminate the significance of the need for social workers in geriatrics in the next century as informed by:

- understanding of the history of the social work profession and its attention to older people and their families;
- knowledge of the current state of geriatric service delivery, social work practice and interdisciplinary teams in the field of aging;
- assessment of the place of geriatrics in the curricula of social work schools and the skills, values, and knowledge that social workers require for effective service delivery and professional practice with older adults;
- assessment of critical issues the profession faces in the changing field of geriatrics;
- vision for the future of social work practice in geriatrics; and therefore
- recommended strategies for the future of social work education and training for that practice.

The first section of this discussion provides a brief description of the history of social work and its relationship to the aging of the population. The second section offers a definition of geriatric social work, key aspects of theory and knowledge base, and settings and systems in which geriatric social work is practiced. In the third section, the best estimates of social workers currently practicing in geriatric systems will be given. Following this brief analysis, attention will turn to describing and analyzing geriatric education and training as it exists today. Then, critical issues in practice, service delivery, and education will follow, with specific attention to the linkages between practice and education. The chapter will conclude with a vision for the future of geriatric social work practice and education, and recommendations for future action required to make that vision a reality.

History of Geriatric Social Work. Lowy wrote in his "Historical Notes on Social Work with the Aging" that "Prior to 1945, not much had been happening in social work with the aging."[1] Compared to the progress that has been made in conceptualization of social work with other populations in medical settings, psychiatric institutions, family service agencies, public welfare departments, etc., and the development of curricula in schools of social work designed to prepare students for practice in these settings, Lowy's conclusion still seems warranted.

But there is another aspect of the history of the social work profession which must be taken into account: from the earliest days, older people as members of families were clients of Charity Organization Societies in many cities, and they were also participants in settlement houses in the neighborhoods where they lived.

Moreover from the day that Richard Cabot appointed Ida Cannon to the staff of the Massachusetts General Hospital, marking the beginning of medical social work, social workers in hospitals have numbered older people among the patients with whom they worked. In the 1930's when Departments of Welfare were established in the states and cities of the country, social workers in these departments had as clients older people receiving Old Age Assistance. In other settings, Veterans Administration facilities, homemaker agencies, mental hospitals and other chronic care facilities, social workers provided services to older people.

The record was not as clear and unambiguous as Lowy's assessment, yet it is patently the case that as the profession developed with its emphasis on the settings and systems in which social workers practiced, aging was not viewed as a specialization nor was there systematic attention to the nature of practice with older people and their families in education of social workers.

It must, of course, be understood that the organization of social service agencies and the nature of social work practice in these agencies and in the health care system were powerfully influenced by the demographic characteristics of the nation. In 1900 when 40% of this population were children under the age of seventeen and only 4% were over the age of 65, or forty years later when 34.4% were under the age of eighteen, and just under 7% were 65 or older, the preoccupation of the profession with children and adolescents and their young or middle-aged parents was understandable. The population was also a great deal more homogeneous, with ethnic minorities making up only a small percentage of the aged persons.

Today with more than 30 million Americans in the 65+ cohort-about one in eight-and with an increase to 54 million, or one in six Americans in this age group, projected for the next quarter of a century, and approximately 12% of those persons being of a minority race or culture, older people are increasingly becoming a focus of the attention of the social work profession. Although, neither practitioners nor administrators, nor academics in the profession can be satisfied with the current state of social work practice in geriatrics or education for that practice.

Moreover, unless strategies and programs are developed now to increase the number of social workers in geriatrics their preparation for careers in geriatrics, the profession will be ill prepared to meet the needs associated with the extraordinary demographic changes.

Social work historically was focused on under-served populations, diversity and community-based care. As in the beginning of the 20th century, the nation is challenged by the need to address increasing diversity with equity. Now in addition, the population as a whole is aging. Social work, which emphasizes working with persons in the community/family context, is key to addressing long-term care needs in a changing health care environment. These foci were never more relevant than now as we enter the next century of geriatric care.

Definition of Geriatric Social Work. First, the matter of terminology and definitions: language will be congruent with the use of the word *geriatric* in the title of this National Forum, but it should be understood that in the profession, social workers may alternatively describe themselves as gerontological social workers or social workers in the field of aging. Geriatrics, in contrast to gerontology, emphasizes practice in health settings with persons in late life or with problems related to aging. Social work practice with older adults is based in mental health and social service settings as well. Geriatric social work, as many of the health professions, is increasingly focused on prevention and wellness in late life as well as problems of aging.

A second point, is the definition of *social work,* and more specifically *geriatric social work.* The National Association of Social Worker's 1981 *Standards for Classification of Social Work Practice* defines social work as[2]:

> *professionally responsible intervention to 1) enhance the developmental, problem solving, and coping capacities of people; 2) promote the effective and humane operating of systems that provide resources and services to people; 3) link people with systems that provide them with resources, services, and opportunities; and 4) contribute to the development and improvement of social policy.*

This definition of the profession permits the geriatric social worker to focus on the strengths and abilities of older people and their families. It calls attention to the important role that social workers play, particularly when the people with whom they work are frail, vulnerable or unfamiliar with service systems, in monitoring the impact of these systems on people, and in helping people secure from service networks the resources they need. The definition reminds us of the responsibility of social workers to participate in the formulation of policies and the design of programs which will benefit older people and their families.

Social Work Theory for Practice: The Bio-Psycho-Social Perspective

Geriatric social work is built on a bio-psycho-social theoretical foundation. The definition of social work includes emphasis on the *person-in-a-socio-cultural-context*, a context which includes the person as a member of a kinship group, a family system, and an informal system which includes neighbors and friends. Coping with illness and disability are viewed within this system's context, which also includes the formal service delivery system and its interaction with informal supports. There is recognition also of differences among ethnic groups in definitions of membership in kinship groups. For example, adoptive kin in many African-American families may be accorded all of the responsibilities and privileges which go with the status of family member. Thus, throughout this chapter, the focus is on geriatric social work *with older people and their families and others in their support systems*.

This perspective provides knowledge for practice which addresses factors that affect normal or *healthy growth and development* in the course of living and includes understanding of the interaction of the biological, psychological, cognitive, and social factors as they affect coping with health and illness. In addition, understanding of family dynamics, knowledge of formal support services and entitlement, awareness of informal care giver stressors and rewards, and the ability to work collaboratively within the continuum of care are essential to successful practice.

The Family Systems Context

In the years following World War II as new suburban communities were being created for young families, sociologists and social workers alike wrote about nuclear families, and either saw older people as isolated from their children and grandchildren or separated by geographic distance and playing relatively minor roles in the lives of the younger members of their families. But in the late 1950's and 1960's, sociologists, Ethel Shanas, Marvin Sussman, and Eugene Litwak among others, began writing about "modified extended families" - family units living separately but linked by bonds of affection and familial responsibility. Older parents maintained their own separate households; adult children moved away; but a shared household was not necessary to the definition of family.[3]

Social work theory and practice, reflecting both the infusion of new understanding about the sociology of families from the social sciences and the experience of social workers in departments of public welfare, family service agencies, and hospitals began to include attention to the role of grandparents in the families. Equally social workers in these settings and also in senior centers were learning about the centrality of family in the lives of older people, and about the extent to which older people relied on the family for emotional support and instrumental help.[4] A growing body of research substantiates the family as the primary source of care in late life, providing over 80% of the support needed by elders.

By the early 1960's, there was a growing body of literature about family relationships and about the necessity for geriatric social workers to recognize families as systems and the family unit, including the elders in it, as the unit of service and treatment.[5] At the same time there was recognition that there were (and are) older people who are kin-less in a functional or absolute sense. Family-less elderly constitute a small minority among the elderly, but it is likely that family-less older people constitute a higher percentage of the clients and patients of geriatric social worker than do the elderly who can rely on their families in time of need.

The recognition of the importance of family systems in the lives of most older people has required that the knowledge base of social work, which has always included systematic and extensive attention to families as social and psychological systems, be expanded to include information about older families and the inter-generational relationships in families, both young and old and their social environments.

The Lifespan Developmental Approach

A second important building block in the knowledge and theory base of social work has been the emphasis on a *lifespan developmental approach* to understand the people geriatric social workers serve. Just as social workers expanded their understanding of families to include older members, friends and neighbors, the knowledge base of the social worker has been enriched in the last several decades by the inclusion of a conceptualization of the tasks, crises and opportunities which characterize the later years of life in the developmental approach. Personality theories of aging which are grounded in this approach include a view of the later years as a time when personal growth and development can continue, rather than as time characterized only by losses, illness and incapacity. The lifespan perspective provides positive goals for social work intervention, with the focus of practice on factors that affect successful aging and normal growth and development in the course of living. Understanding the intersection of biological, psychological, sociocultural, and economic factors which affect normal growth and development in the course of living is required, as well as an understanding of the interaction of these factors.

The developmental approach requires of social workers that they take into careful account the individual and family histories of the people whom they serve. The developmental approach also obliges geriatric social workers to understand and accredit the strengths of the individuals and family as a system, and the "stresses and presses" which they experience. Central to the lifespan development approach are two key concepts — *coping* and *adaptation.* If older people, facing the problems of the later years, can be helped by the social worker to identify coping strategies that have served them well when they were younger, they may then be able to claim their earlier competencies and to again make effective use of these strategies. Understanding the *adaptation* process will help the social worker to see that what looks like irrational behavior may represent the older person's effort to adapt to what *was*, rather than what *is*.

Cohort theory is also key to the life span developmental approach; that is, it is important for social workers to know about the cohort of the older people with whom they work, the unique social context into which the members of the cohort were born, grew up, were adults, and are now growing older.

Recognition of Ethnic Diversity and Special Populations

The recognition of the socio-cultural heterogeneity of the older population of the United States is a relatively recent addition to the intellectual foundation of gerontology.[6] The extraordinary diversity of this population creates complex problems in the development and delivery of health and social services to older Americans, and places demands on the geriatric social worker. Diversity in this context refers to minority groups in the older population—

African-Americans, American Indians/Alaskan Natives, Asian/Pacific Islanders, and Hispanic Americans, whose life histories and situations in old age are powerfully affected by the "presses" they have experienced. Many have lived lives blighted by discrimination, poverty and poor functional health status. Their health beliefs and health care practices are grounded in their sociocultural and ethnic backgrounds,[7] and competent geriatric social workers understand and respect these beliefs and practices.

It is essential that geriatric social workers understand the full dimensions of the ethnic diversity of the elderly population. Now the non-white group among the elderly is growing rapidly, and before the mid point of the next century, approximately 20% of the older population will be non-white.[8]

Significant differences between ethnic groups are found in life-expectancy and economic status. There is also great variation within each of the minority groupings in culture, language, national origin, religion, health practice and belief.[9]

Native Americans are the smallest minority group and they have the smallest percentage of elders in their population. Native American aged persons have the lowest life expectancy, highest rates of poverty, and extremely high rates of poor health. African Americans are the second longest minority residents in this country and have the largest group of seniors who enter old age after a lifetime of legal discrimination, social and economic deprivation, poor health services, high rates of poor health and chronic disease.[10]

Although Hispanic persons have been in the United States for more than two hundred years, their numbers and needs were largely overlooked until the 1960's. Similar to all the other minority groups, persons designated as Hispanic come from a number of different countries and regions of the world and differ widely in their levels of economic well being, acculturation, and health practices. Many older Hispanics, however, prefer to speak Spanish, continue to use native healers, and maintain health beliefs and practices that differ from other minorities and the majority group (SGEC Working Papers, 1989).

Due to the history of Asians in this country and specific immigration laws limiting their admittance to their country, the profile of their numbers, gender, and length of time is different from other minority groups. Asian elders are the only group of elders in which the number of males outnumbers the females. They also have the largest number of foreign-born elders coming to the U.S. as political refugees or emigrating from territories that are protectorates of the U.S.[11]

The older population in the United States includes other groups that require specific knowledge, sensitivity and interventions by geriatric social workers. These groups include persons with alternate life styles, e.g., gay or lesbian persons, persons with specific religions that require different practices than our majority culture, and persons with developmental disabilities or health problems. Yet another factor of diversity in our older population is the length of this age period which contains persons of several different generations and co-host groupings. The knowledge base of geriatric social workers must include understanding of the differences in the problems and challenges faced by 65-year olds and 85-year olds—all members of the older population, but at very different stages of their life cycles, and with different psycho-social needs.

Finally, there are those elderly with special needs based in diseases, illnesses, or social problems which may carry shame, stigma, and disapproval from American society. Included are persons suffering from HIV/AIDS, alcoholism, drug addiction, mental illness, and other diseases which are viewed by many Americans as the results of deviant behaviors. Geriatric social workers need to include questions in their assessment interviews with all older adults which will reveal if they have a problem with one or more of these diseases or conditions. In addition, it is important that geriatric social workers exercise considerable caution in the selection and use of standard screening measures. Many such measures yield flawed or misleading results. Unless geriatric social workers limit the use of screening measures for such problems as alcoholism to those measures that have proven valid for use with elderly persons or have been developed specifically for use with these persons, there is a risk of misinterpreting the results, which often leads to inaccurate assessments and unsuccessful outcomes.

Current Status of Geriatric Social Work: Geriatric Social Work Settings and Systems

Settings

In addition to the diversity of the population of older people who come to the health and social service system, account must also be taken of the diversity of services and systems. Service diversity includes the particular societal task assignments of the agencies and institutions which constitute the systems, the differences in the ways they are staffed and organized, and the way(s) in which the role of the social worker is specified.

Given this diversity it is clear that the preparation of social work students for geriatric practice must include attention to the history of these systems and settings. Course work needs to include organizational analysis and the sociology of formal organizations and professional practice, as well as the place and work of the social worker in various settings.

The health and social service settings and systems for geriatric social worker practice include:

- General and Specialized Hospitals, including Mental Hospitals
- Health Care Clinics, Ambulatory Care, Community Mental Health Centers, and Family Services
- Home Health Care Agencies
- The Department of Veterans Affairs, VA Medical Centers
- Independent physicians' and dentists' practices
- Nursing Homes and Hospices
- Managed Care
- Adult Day Care and Respite programs
- Geriatric Case Management agencies or private practices
- Senior Centers and Nutrition Programs/Information and Referral
- Senior Citizens apartments, Assisted Living Programs and Public Housing Projects
- Area Agencies on Aging and social service and health planning agencies
- Agencies in the Mental Retardation/Developmentally Disabled network, serving older people with developmental disabilities and their families
- Legal Service Agencies
- Departments of Public Welfare/Social Services
- Agencies serving older Gays and Lesbians and agencies serving people with HIV/AIDS
- Child Welfare Agencies,serving children being cared for by their

grandparents or other older relatives
- Agencies and institutions in substance dependency networks
- Employees Assistance Programs in corporations and in unions

In all of these settings social workers' goals include helping older people maintain their autonomy and independence, helping them to live, even when faced with increased disability and loss. Thus the preparation of the geriatric social workers must include attention to benefits, entitlements, and other community resources available to older people and their families, and training in system linkages.

Interdisciplinary Teamwork

The inter-relationship of social, psychological, biological, and economic factors in determining the situations of older people and the nature of their need for help makes a team approach to professional practice and service delivery essential. Educational needs of students preparing for careers as geriatric social workers include an emphasis on the skills, knowledge, and values required for effective team work.

Social workers are key members of the interdisciplinary team required to deal with complex problems of older persons. In the early 1900's, the social worker joined with the doctor and the nurse to compose the inpatient care team.[12] By the turn of the century, social work had developed as a health-related profession offering services to meet a variety of psychological, social and environmental needs. Following the passage of the Social Security amendments of 1935, problems in coordination of care increased. Social work was perceived as the major linkage between medical and environmental resources.

Interdisciplinary teamwork recognizes that the complexities of old people's problems necessitate a comprehensive and planned approach to their resolution. Interdisciplinary teamwork benefits the elderly person in terms of coordinated service, more skilled services, avoidance of duplication of services, the introduction of preventive services, and convenience, not burdening the client with integrating needed services.

Social Work Case Management

From the early beginnings of the profession, the definition of social work has always included responsibility for what is now called case management, that is, the responsibility to secure the resources older adults need in a timely and appropriate fashion, and for facilitating the linkages among agencies and systems in order to ensure continuity of services. Today, case management is an essential component of the provision of care to older people, partly because of the fragmentation and discontinuities in the service delivery system, and partly because of the emphasis on cost efficiency and effectiveness. Although other professions are engaged in the provision of case management, the expertise of geriatric social workers continues to be a strong justification for the centrality of their role as case managers, and for this being part of their assignments on geriatric interdisciplinary teams. In the next decade, the social work practice of case management will be refined on the basis of data about the outcomes experienced by patients receiving long term care in the community.

Current and Projected Labor Force

There is a clear linkage between the present and projected increase in the number of older people in the United States and in the increasing demand for health and social services for this population, and, therefore, the labor market demand for geriatric social workers. Projections of the need for geriatric social workers[13, 14] have consistently and significantly exceeded the number of social workers being educated in the professional schools and universities of our nation.

According to the U.S. Bureau of Labor Statistics (BLS), there were 484,178 Americans employed in social work positions in 1992, and the BLS predicts that by the year 2005, that number will increase by 191,372 to 675,547—an approximate 40% increase in just 13 years.[15] It must be understood that these are aggregate figures which do not provide data about the educational preparation or settings in which these social workers practice.

Social work employment can also be assessed through analysis of information about the membership of the National Association of Social Workers (NASW), the largest organization of professional social workers in the world. The NASW data have the advantage of providing information about the educational level of its members, but it must be understood that not all practicing social workers are NASW members. To illustrate: in 1991 NASW's membership was 134,240, in comparison with the 484,178 identified by the BLS in 1992 as holders of social work titles.[15, 16] NASW studies, however, do yield data about the members' education and practice areas. In 1991 7.4% of NASW members had bachelor's degrees; the vast majority of the NASW membership, 87.5%, had earned their Master's Degrees, and 4.7% had completed their doctoral work.[16] Clearly underrepresented in the NASW membership are social workers with bachelor's degrees, for it is known that the majority of social workers in the labor force are baccalaureate graduates, not holders of graduate degrees.

With respect to primary practice areas, 12.7% of NASW members with bachelor's degrees identified aging as their practice area; as did 4.2% of the M.S.W.'s, and an equal percentage of the D.S.W.'s.[16] Only a little over 5% identify aging as primary practice (Figure 3.1). A total of 10.5% (or 7,900) of the NASW membership, regardless of educational level, identified aging as their primary or secondary area of practice.[16] However, more than a third (36.2%) of the NASW members listed hospitals or medical clinics as the settings in which they are employed, and it is safe to assume that a majority of their clients include older people[16] (see Figure 3.2).

The wide variety of settings in which significant numbers of social workers practice was noted in the first section of this chapter. Thus, it can be concluded that available data clearly and substantially underestimate the number of social workers whose practice includes work with older people and their families, although aging may not be viewed as the workers' primary practice area.

Current Social Work Education and Training

NASW reports that geriatric social work is among the fastest growing specializations within the profession, and further that regardless of the specialization or the setting in which the social work is practicing, 62% of NASW members report that geriatric knowledge is required in their position.[17] Given the changing age character of the American population, and the importance which practicing social workers attach to knowledge about the process of aging and older people, what is the current state of geriatric education in social work?

Between 1989 and 1993, the number of Accredited Master's Degree Programs and Doctoral Programs increased from 97 to 111 and from 47 to 53 respectively according to the *Council of Social Work Education (CSWE), the accrediting body for social work education in the United States*. The number of Baccalaureate programs in 1989 was unchanged in 1993, remaining at 242.

To assess geriatric social work education, data was taken from the 1988 and 1994 national surveys done by the Social Work Faculty Development Program (SWFDP) of the California Geriatric Education Center at UCLA, findings of which were compared with those generated in earlier studies of social work education.

Though employment data reveal that many geriatric social work positions are held by people with a B.A. degree only, and so the 1988 CGEC finding that 80% of the Baccalaureate programs provide no course work in aging is particularly disquieting.[18] In 11% of these programs some geriatric course work is offered, and only 9% offer their students the opportunity for a concentration in aging.[18]

The picture in Master's Degree programs is more encouraging: the number of schools offering specialized concentrations in aging increased from 33% in 1988 to 39% in 1994, and the number of schools reporting no course work in aging decreased during that period from 33% to 23%.[18, 19] In 1994 an additional 35% of the schools reported some aging content course work in their courses (see Figure 3.1). Thus almost three quarters of the schools offer at least some geriatric education in the classroom. The vast majority of schools have field opportunities to work with older people and their families.

The number of schools that offer course work in aging is only one measure of the adequacy of the profession's response to the need for increasing numbers of well educated geriatric social workers. Questions must also be posed about the level of curriculum development in the schools. Damron-Rodriguez and Lubben[20] have suggested six criteria to be used as the measure of curricula development level. These are delineated in Table 3.1.

The criteria are used to distinguish two levels of curricula adoption: (1) minimal aging content integration and (2) substantial aging curricula development, with the substantial level characterized by structural changes in the school curriculum and significant commitment of resources to geriatric course work and field experience. In 1988, based on these criteria, 58% of the schools met the minimum standards, and in 32%, there was evidence of substantial development in geriatric education.[18] Analyses of 1994 data based on these criteria show an increase in schools of social work meeting both minimal and substantial criteria.[20] In 1994, 74% of graduate schools met minimal criteria but less than one half (40%) substantially met criteria for gerontological curricula. More extensive analysis of the data yields the inescapable conclusion that despite progress in terms of the number of schools in which there is geriatric course content in the curricula, there is much work to be done, particularly in increasing the number of classroom and field faculty with substantial expertise in geriatric social work, and the number of students enrolled in aging courses and/or placed in clinical practice sites offering substantial opportunity to work with older people and their families. In 1988, only 3% of the graduating MSW students had taken a gerontology social work course. That number increased to 5% in 1994. Of special importance is the necessity to recruit more students and faculty from minority communities, to develop more field instruction centers in these communities, and in systems serving special populations of older people.

Gerontological content areas have been identified for the foundation-level course curriculum in graduate social work education and include the 14 aging-related topics and 12 aging-related skill areas originally described in the Gerontological Society of America and the Association of Gerontology in Higher Education project funded by the Administration on Aging.[20] These areas were selected based on a consensus of social work educators in aging as composing the essential components of gerontology in the MSW program. There is a growing consensus since initial work of what constitutes the core knowledge base, attitudes and skills for work with older adults and their families.[14, 17, 21, 22]

Examination of the current state of geriatric education and training must also focus on specific content areas which are essential to the knowledge base of the geriatric social worker. In the introductory section to this chapter, some elements of the theory and knowledge foundation of geriatric social work were provided, including the emphasis on a life span approach; on understanding the family relationships of older people, and their role and status in kinship groups; on knowledge about the settings and systems in which geriatric social workers practice, and the requirements for interdisciplinary teamwork; on familiarity with benefits and entitlements and other resources, and on the demands on social workers imposed by their roles in advocacy and system linkage, etc. The critical importance of the geriatric social worker's knowledge of and respect for the diversity of the older population of the United States was emphasized.

Curricula content having to do with *special populations of older people* is so critical that it merits special attention here. CSWE pioneered in efforts (funded primarily by the Administration on Aging) to address the need to include in the school curricula specific content about minority elderly. However, progress in making changes in this curriculum area have been slow. Students continue to graduate without achieving sufficient knowledge about the socio-cultural backgrounds of the older people with whom they work, including understanding of language, idioms, and special expressions, for example; about the particular obstacles and difficulties which may prevent older people in minority communities from gaining access to the resources and services they need.[23, 24, 25]

Funding for Geriatric Social Work Education

Clearly, consideration of recommendations for strategic directions for the future of geriatric education for social workers requires that the resources available in support of that education be identified, as well as the needs and tasks which must claim the attention of this funding for gerontological education has historically come from four major sources:

- federal agencies;
- philanthropic foundations;
- stipends provided by local agencies, both voluntary and public, which serve as field instruction centers for the schools, and
- the internal resources of the academic institutions in which social work education schools and programs are located.

Federal agencies have played a key role in

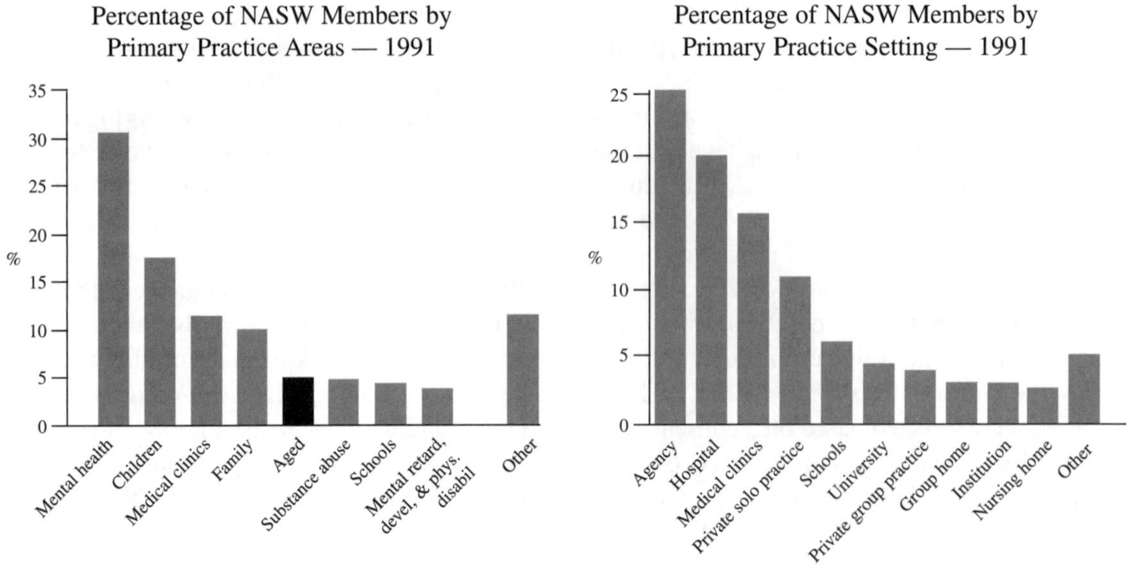

Figure 3.1 (Data taken from Giblmam & Schervich, 1993)

support of geriatric education in social work, particularly the Bureau of Health Professions, Veterans Administration, the Administration on Aging, and the Center for Mental Health Services of Health and Human Services. The following section offers a brief presentation of the activities of each of these four federal agencies.

The Health Resources and Services Administration (HRSA), Bureau of Health Professions. A major new initiative in geriatric education was launched by the Health Resources and Services Administration (HRSA) in 1984, with the establishment of the first four HRSA-funded Geriatric Education Centers (GEC). The GEC program was designed as a strategy to increase the number of faculty in Schools of Medicine, Nursing, Allied Health, Dentistry, Social Work, etc., who had expertise in and a commitment to geriatrics. Of central importance in the program was the emphasis on the engagement of the medical schools of the nation in preparation of physicians and other health professionals for geriatric practice. In addition, the design of the program required that the curricula of all of the GECs include content which would help faculty in all professional schools to prepare their students for their roles on interdisciplinary teams.

In the years since 1984, GECs have been founded, and the National Association of Geriatric Education Centers includes in its membership *both* currently funded GECs (20 in Fiscal Year 1994) and Centers which no longer have HRSA funding, but which have maintained their programs with funds from other sources. There are a total of 45 GECs presently active. Of the 20 currently funded, 16 include social work among the professions for which geriatric educational experiences are being provided.

Analysis of the programs of the GECs provides evidence of the extraordinary diversity of the educational programs offered by the Centers. And it should be noted that early on in many of the social

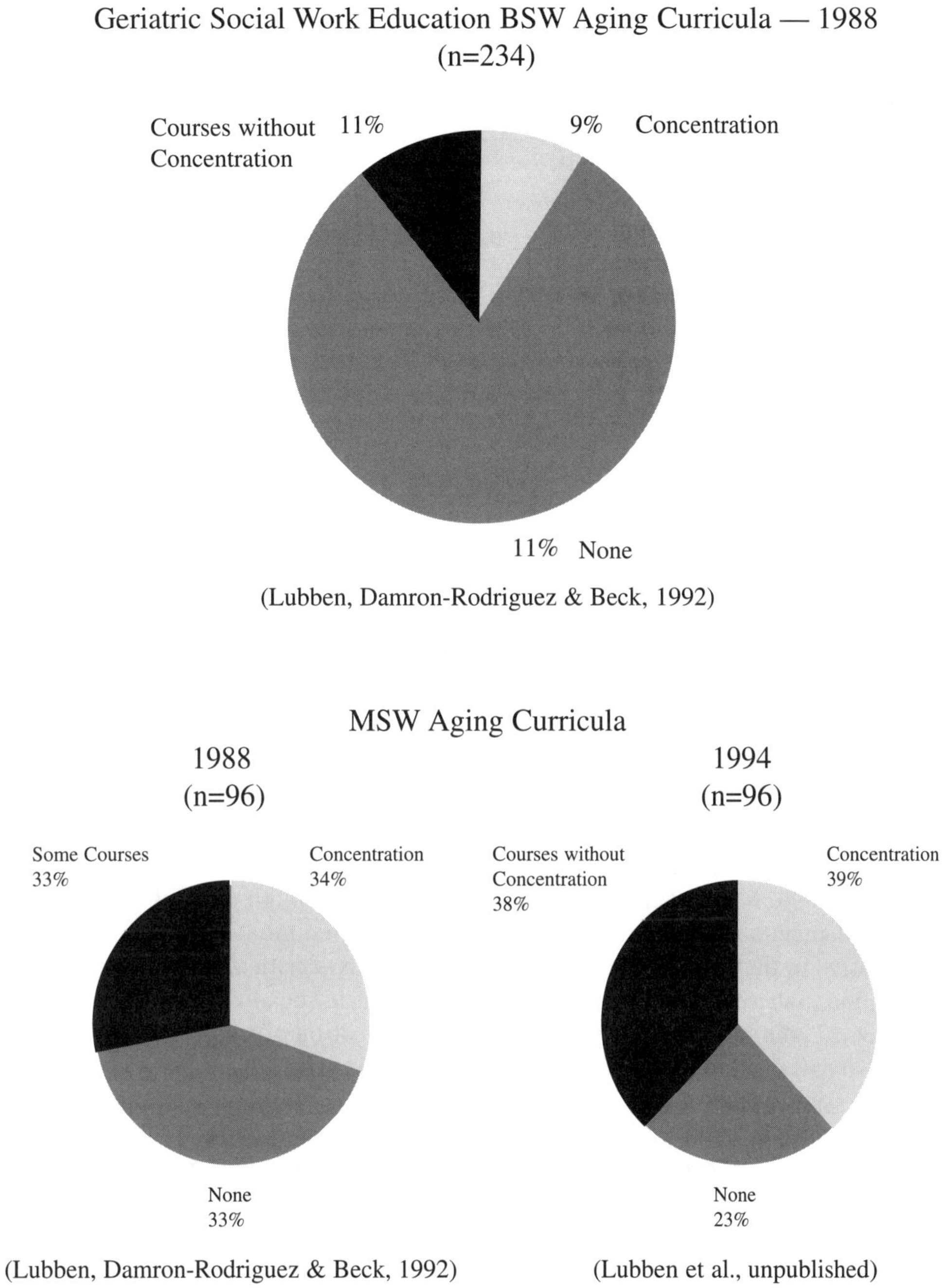
Geriatric Social Work Education BSW Aging Curricula — 1988
(n=234)
Courses without Concentration 11%
9% Concentration
11% None
(Lubben, Damron-Rodriguez & Beck, 1992)
MSW Aging Curricula
1988
(n=96)
Some Courses 33%
Concentration 34%
None 33%
(Lubben, Damron-Rodriguez & Beck, 1992)
1994
(n=96)
Courses without Concentration 38%
Concentration 39%
None 23%
(Lubben et al., unpublished)

Figure 3.2

Table 3.1 Percentage of Programs Meeting Minimal and Substantial Criteria for Gerontological Curriculum Development (N=97), 1994[20]

Criteria	MINIMAL Standard	%	SUBSTANTIAL Standard	%
Number of courses	1–2 Elective	78%	3+ Required	17%
Number of students in aging	Any students?	68%	5% of students	46%
Stability:				
Number of students in 3+ years	1 or more students	73%	5% of students	50%
Faculty in aging	Any - full or part time	63%	1 or more full time	61%
Field faculty in aging	Any - full or part time	73%	1 or more full time	67%
Field placement sites	2 sites	96%	4+ sites	91%
Composite adoption measure	4 or more standards	74%	4 or more standards	40%

work programs, geriatric social workers in the field who carry major in-service training and supervision responsibilities in their agencies and institutions were included, along with school of social work faculty, as enrollees and participants in the educational programs of the GECs. The target group of the GECs are academics and trainers who are enrollees in the GEC program, who will complete at least 40 hours of training, and who will implement a new geriatric educational initiative in their school or agency. But in addition to these enrollees, of which there were 30,272 during the years 1984–93, there are also participants in the GEC programs, professionals and faculty who are invited to attend GEC's educational offerings, but who are not enrolled for the full program. In this time period (1984–93), there are 195,163 professional participants in GECs in this fashion.

During these years geriatric social workers comprised 21.3% of all the enrollees, and 11.3% of all participants; 6,441 social workers were in the first category, and 21,933 were participants. The nursing profession ranked first in number and percent of both participants and enrollees, accounting for approximately 25% of the professionals in each category. Medicine ranked second in the number and percent of participants (31,756, amounting to 16.3%), but ranked third, behind both social work and nursing in the number and percent of enrollees.

Thus, although the GECs are not social work degree granting programs, many of these play a critical role in the preparation of geriatric social work faculty, and also in the education of training staff in the field. The 6441 enrollees in the years since 1984 represent a critical mass and provide at least a partial solution to the problem of the shortage of geriatric social work faculty.

The Department of Veterans Affairs. Historically there has been an ebb and flow to the support provided by federal agencies. Only the Department of Veterans Affairs (VA) has been able to maintain a stable level of support for social work education in general and gerontological education in particular. In part, the stability of VA support can be accounted for through an examination of the history of the four agencies: VA is, of course, the oldest of the four, and its mission of service to American veterans and their families has always included responsibility for the clinical education of professionals for VA and the nation.

The VA was one of the first federal programs to take initiative in geriatric training and education. VA strength in geriatrics is founded in the recognition of the rapid aging of the veteran population. Of the 27 million veterans in 1994, 31% are over the age of 65. By the 2015 nearly 50% of veterans will be over 65 years of age.

As will be seen, during the past ten-year period, 1149 candidates for the M.S.W. degree received VA support for geriatric clinical experiences, and, excluding the year 1986 when for idiosyncratic reasons VA was able to award 204 stipends to M.S.W. candidates, the numbers are remarkably stable, ranging from a low in 1990 of 98 to a high of 118 in 1995, with the average being 105. In addition, on average VA each year funds 300 clinical placements for second year students, and these are above and beyond the 1149.

VA also provides support for M.S.W. candidates through other programs. This year, for example, 84 students are receiving VA stipends through the Primary Care Education Program, and in addition there is funding support for clinical educational experiences for social work students in the Geriatric Research, Education and Clinical Centers (GRECCs), of which there are 16 located at 18 VAMCs. In all, VA is presently supporting the clinical education experiences of 400 M.S.W. candidates. Moreover, there are twelve VAMCs located across the country which host Interdisciplinary Team Training programs in which social workers and other professionals are educated for the team approach to treatment, an approach central to the work of the VAs.

Analysis of funding for professional education in the Department of Veterans Affairs has probably been less contingent on specific and changing priorities in the Congress, and, therefore, more stable. In 1994 alone, 211 multidisciplinary trainees (72 were social workers) were supported at 71 VA medical centers at a cost of $1,813, 918. The Associated Health in Geriatrics Traineeship Program remains a special priority in the VA Office of Academic Affairs and has continued to be an expanding program. Of the total VA 1994 training funds $3237,202 were committed to the training of 508 health professional students with 115 of the trainees being social workers (Office of Academic Affairs, 1994). Current geriatric social work stipends for students are approximately $3,800 a year.

A key educational opportunity for social work students was the establishment of the Geriatric Research, Education and Clinical Centers (GRECCs) to integrate research education and model clinical services. There are currently 16 GRECCs providing an interdisciplinary approach to geriatric training with social work being a core discipline. Additionally, in 12 VAMCs where GRECCs are not located, there are Inter-Disciplinary Team Training Programs (ITTP) in which social workers and other professionals are educated for the team approach to treatment. In 1995, for example, 84 students are receiving VA stipends through the Primary Care Education Program (PRIME).

VA includes research as an integral part of geriatric training particularly at the doctoral and postdoctoral levels. GRECC provides research mentors and other research support. VA has a national research program with annual funding of more than $200 million and a significant portion of the research is related to geriatrics.[24] Increasingly, research is an integral part of VA social work education.[26]

The Administration on Aging. The Older Americans Act, which established the Administration on Aging (AoA), was passed in 1965, and from the beginning,

> *The Administration on Aging assumed that it was the intent of the Congress to provide support for training professional and technical personnel for service primarily in newly emergent occupations which have come into existence in response to the needs of the older population and for which training support had not been available under existing grant programs. . . . Education and training in aging . . . have been increasing during recent years . . . particularly . . . for professional practice in public health, nursing, psychiatry, clinical psychology, social work, and vocational rehabilitation. (emphasis added).*[20]

It is clear from these and other documents that the original goals for the implementation of the Older Americans Act including preparation of students in a variety of professions, including social work, for careers in gerontology and geriatrics. It was not possible to secure hard data about AoA funding levels of social work education, or estimates of the number of M.S.W. candidates receiving AoA provided stipends. However, an examination of an *AoA Compendium of Grants*[3] provides evidence of some grants specifically designed to support social work education programs, and many more in which social workers were included among the targeted trainees. It appears that during the early years of the Administration, roughly 1965–1980, there was considerable AOA support for entry-level and advanced education in gerontological and geriatric professions, and that social work was central in many of these AoA supported educational programs.[4]

In the year 1980, however, funding for Title IV projects has declined, and in the words of Edward F. Ansello, testifying in his role as President of the Association for Gerontology in Higher Education before the Subcommittee on Human Services of the U.S. House of Representatives Select Committee on Aging in 1990,

> *In recent years Title IV's focus has become more blurred. The emphasis upon social . . . aspects of aging has been diluted by increasing attention to biomedical issues. . . . Further, the balance among the Title's basic components has been shifted, with a dramatic de-emphasis of education and research.*[5]

The combination of the decline in Title IV funding and the changes in priorities for the use of available funds undoubtedly accounts for the decline in the last 15 years of AoA funding for social work education. In comparison with the first 15 years of AoA, fewer distinctly social work projects have been funded, and more characteristically, if funds are allocated for professional education initiatives, social work may be one of several professions included in a program. In the *Compendium* issued in January, 1988, and cited above, for example, 274 grants were identified of which *three* were in support of social work education, and a number of others, particularly for in-service training and continuing education initiatives, included social workers among the staff to be trained.

It appears possible that during Fiscal Year

1996 there will be modest funding of traditional university-based career training initiatives. If this proves to be the case, then social work education at the Master's level may be among the beneficiaries of this initiative.

The Center for Mental Health Services, NIMH. The National Institute of Mental Health has for many years been an important source of support for social work education programs. From the 1950's, to '70's, annual budgets for NIMH-sponsored clinical training programs were 90 million dollars. One-fourth of the students being supported in these programs were social work students. In 1980, however, the allocation for clinical training projects dropped to 70 million dollars, and in 1986, the reduction was to 20 million.

Table 3.2 is included in this Report with permission of the Center of Mental Health Services, National Institute of Mental Health.[27] It gives a picture of the important role the Center played in the period 1992–94, a period in which almost 200 social work students received support for their studies. For 156 of these students, almost 8%, "Elderly with Mental Disorders" was identified as their "primary priority population." The conclusion is inescapable that the Center and the Training Branch which carried the mental health clinical training responsibilities prior to the establishment of the Center were key sources of support for social work education.[27] A conference convened by the Center in February, 1993 was devoted to a discussion of "Workforce Training and Development for Mental Health Systems." The Report includes attention to "priority needs" and a series of recommendations directed to "the academic community, the public mental health system, and for CMHS." It also includes a summary of funding of mental health clinic training from the year 1948 through 1993, another indicator of the importance of the CMHS and its predecessor agencies.[28]

The current picture is, however, a bleak one. The last grants for social work students were given in September, 1994, and there are presently no funds available for support of new grants.

It should be noted also that the Mental Disorders of the Aging Research Branch did provide limited support for social work education at the Master's Level in the 1960's and '70's. The work of the Branch is now entirely focused on research, and it carries no training responsibilities.

Mention should also be made of the National Institute on Aging. The NIA has never been a significant source of support for social work education at either the Master's or the Doctoral level. However, during the past ten years, NIA has supported a doctoral and post-doctoral training grant at the School of Social Work, University of Michigan. The annual amount of the grant is approximately $460,000.00, and the purpose is to support the development of social work resin geriatrics and gerontology.

Critical Issues in Geriatric Social Work

A number of significant issues in geriatric education for social workers must be considered if a sufficient number of competent and committed social workers are to be prepared for practice with older people and their families. These issues must be confronted by the profession in the context of the extraordinary changes which are occurring in the health and social service systems and in the settings in which geriatric social workers practice. Note must be taken of the

- emphasis on managed care strategies designed to contain health care costs and rationalize the system, and the key role that social workers are being called upon to play as case managers;

- increasing emphasis on community based geriatric services, outside the walls of hospitals and long-term care facilities, an emphasis which underscores the importance of the preparation of geriatric social workers for work with families; for system linkage and advocacy roles, etc.;
- on-going debate about the role of government in meeting the health and social service needs of the citizenry, and the increasing emphasis on the public-private partnership and the role of voluntary agencies in the provision of services;
- move toward a devolution of responsibilities for health and social services from the federal government to state and local governments, and toward block grants, replacing the programmatic funding of many service areas;
- move toward continuous quality improvement evaluation of program changes, increased necessity for data collection and program and practice accountability;
- change and demographics which demonstrate dramatically the need for geriatric social work to respond to the increasing percentage of minority aged, diversity of life styles and specific populations aged persons with diseases of stigma, elders with different levels of acculturation, income and education that impact access and needs for services;
- lag in social work licensing laws to respond to the needs for protection of consumers by assurance of knowledgeable and skilled geriatric social workers by revised content in the examination and demonstrated by passage of the content in the revised tests for licensure;
- critical need to address the downward spiral of salaries to make geriatric social workers most attractive as a field of study and employment;
- lack of responsiveness of schools of social work to change curriculum content, of faculty to develop expertise in geriatrics and of the accrediting body to encourage, support, or pressure the schools into making the needed adjustments.

To discuss the implications of these and other trends and changes which are occurring in the body politic is beyond the ken of this chapter. All of the service delivery, practice, and educational issues faced by social workers are powerfully affected by events in Washington, our state capitols, and our city halls.

Curriculum Design. Schools of medicine, nursing, health sciences and of social work share curriculum issues. Should geriatric content be integrated in all courses where it is relevant and appropriate or should there be a specialized geriatric educational track?

Level of Education Required for Geriatric Social Work. This Report's discussion of the current state of geriatric education in social work noted the three levels of social work education, baccalaureate (BSW), graduate (MSW), and doctoral (Ph.D or DSW). Given the three levels of education, there are on-going issues facing the profession and the agencies in which geriatric social workers practice having to do with definition of the educational credentials for different positions. In the schools there is the need for clear distinctions in content range and complexity in the three levels.

Table 3.2 Priority Populations Served in Payback Service, by Number of Trainees and Months of Service Provided: Social Work*

	Trainees**		Months	
	N	%	N	%
Total Trainees	1,967	100.0	***	100.0
Minorities with Mental Disorders	409	20.8	13.739	21.6
Children & Adolescents with Mental Disorders	413	21.0	9,788	15.4
Poverty Populations with Mental Disorders	296	15.0	11,206	17.6
Seriously Mentally Ill Adults	243	12.3	5,928	9.3
Substance Abusers	100	5.1	5,476	8.6
Individuals with Mental Disorders in Rural Areas	65	3.3	1,686	2.6
All Others	156	7.9	4,549	7.1
	286	14.5	11,336	17.8

* Total number, as of March 25, 1993.

** Trainees are unduplicated. When a trainee had more than one priority population, his/her primary priority population was used for classification purposes.

*** Month categories may overlap, so month total is not meaningful.

Center for Mental Health Services, SAMHSA

The Educational Barriers to Progress. As future directions are charted, issues must be faced having to do with the obstacles which have stood in the way of more rapid progress of geriatric social work curriculum. In 1988, the lack of *faculty* with expertise in geriatrics was cited as a major barrier in the development of geriatric education in social work. In 1994, four major barriers were identified: the *fiscal constraints* under which most schools operate (41%) and which limit the recruitment of faculty expert in geriatrics and the development and offering of new courses; *student resistance* (28%) and the view of older people as a *low priority population* (19%) and lack of trained faculty (17%) (19). The interconnections among these barriers are clear: when many faculty and students share a negative view of geriatric social work practice and when there are few or no faculty who claim geriatric social work as their primary field of practice and when there are limited funds available for expansion and recruitment, progress is difficult and slow.

Geriatric Social Work Salaries. One such strategy has to do with salary scales in the field. Social work with the aged was the identified as the lowest paying primary area of practice for NASW members in 1991, with a mean annual salary of $24,332.00.[26] Clearly so long as social work practice with older people in senior centers, in community based home care and case management agencies, etc. is known to be poorly paid in comparison with other settings and systems, student resistance and the low priority assigned to geriatric social work are difficult barriers to overcome and issues to resolve.

It should be noted here that field training sites exist for all schools in rich abundance - testimony to the variety of roles for geriatric social workers and the increasing professionalization of geriatric social work practice in recent years.

Education for Diversity. Education must take account of the increasing diversity in the older population of the United States, a diversity that includes differences in ethnic and socio-cultural backgrounds and heritages, and special needs and strengths. It was noted that some of these special needs are associated with life styles and health conditions, and also noted was the presence in the aging population of two generations or more who are at different states in their life cycle. There are several critical issues to be faced in order to ensure that our social work students achieve the knowledge, values, and skills required for competent geriatric social work practice with these diverse groups of older people and their families, and other members of their support systems, particularly friends and neighbors.

The barriers already discussed impinge powerfully on the capacities of Schools of Social Work to recruit faculty who have the expertise and experience to teach about these diverse groups; to interest students in careers serving these populations, particularly students who themselves come from minority or disadvantaged communities.

Informal Support Systems of Older People. Central to curricula is the need to emphasize geriatric social work practice and service delivery to older people *and their families and other members of their support systems.* Again the location of content in the curriculum is an issue to be faced. Is specialized course work required for students planning for careers as geriatric social workers?

Diverse Practice Settings and Systems. The general/specific issue is also important in consideration of the need of geriatric social workers for understanding of the various settings and systems to which older people and their families come for help.

The need for geriatric social work should be defined by practice with or in behalf of older adults and their families regardless of setting and population designation. Settings that serve significant numbers of older persons require health care practitioners, social workers included, to be educationally prepared to meet their needs. The practitioner may identify as a medical social worker or mental health clinician but if the clientele is aged then there is a need for a knowledge base in aging. Social work labor, education and training must continuously change to relate to new arenas of care (i.e. home care, assisted living, managed care).

The Developmental Life Span Approach. The developmental life span approach requires systematic attention to the later years of life in courses in the Human Behavior and Social Environment sequence. Issues having to do with faculty expertise and commitment to sufficient coverage of the later years in these courses must be resolved, and the connections between the aging content included in required courses, and that to be included in specialized geriatric courses need to be made and articulated.

Interdisciplinary Team Education. Issues to be raised: at what point in the educational program should there be classroom content about the team approach? How do school and field faculty collaborate to design opportunities in the field for students to participate in multidisciplinary teams? How do school and field faculty ensure that students are helped to feel comfortable and secure *as social workers* while, at the same time, learning about and learning to respect the work of other members of the team?

To conclude: the claim cannot be made that *all* of the critical issues which social work educators face in the charting of the future direction of education for geriatric practice have been discussed in this section. The attempt has been to identify priority issues which require immediate and ongoing attention, and which seem crucial to efforts to ensure that both numerical and competency goals are met in the years ahead.

Continuous Quality Improvement. The Pew Foundation has been a leader in recommendations for health professional education reform.[27] Key issues for their recommendations relate to the need to monitor and evaluate practice in order to be accountable as professionals and to overseeing agents. This approach requires technological skills in data management and an intervention research approach. This continuous quality improvement perspective is needed as well in addressing change in social work curriculum and accountability for educational outcomes.

Vision for Geriatric Social Work Education and Practice

The demographic revolution makes changes in social work education for geriatric practice an imperative. Geriatric social work must envision service delivery and professional practice to assure the needs of those who will grow older in the 21st Century are met in a timely and appropriate fashion, and that the diverse older population will live productive, secure and dignified lives.

1. The vision is for an *integrated health and social service system* in which boundaries are no longer obstacles in the path between older people and the services they need, and the boundaries are no longer there to protect professional or organizational turf.

2. The vision includes systems and settings in which the *life histories and sociocultural, religious, ethnic, and life style backgrounds of older people are understood and respected*, and which there is open and equal access for all. It is envisioned that social workers in these agencies represent the diversity of ethnicity, life styles, sociocultural backgrounds, and health statuses of the elderly they serve. This envisions *all staff, regardless of background and orientation, achieve knowledge, values, and skills necessary to work effectively with older people.*

3. The vision is for agencies and institutions to *be located in facilities which are easily accessible to older people*, including those who are frail or disabled.

4. The vision is for social workers to work to *ensure the autonomy of older people and their participation in decisions and plans for them.* This envisions *a partnership between the professional and the older person* and that family members receive the help they need to remain supportive to their elders.

5. The vision emphases linkages with *self-help and mutual aid groups and activities*, so that social workers help older people to be empowered and encouraged to take responsibility for themselves and at the same time to help other age peers find solutions to the life cycle problems and challenges they face, and find fulfillment in the later years.

6. The vision includes *health and social services being delivered by members of interdisciplinary teams on which social*

workers play a key role, with the teams characterized by respectful and cooperative relationships among the members.

7. This envisions *geriatric social workers in a variety of different roles:* as clinicians working directly with older people and their families; as care coordinators and case managers, making certain that the resources needed are in fact available; as administrators of agencies and institutions; as planners and policy makers; as teachers and researchers.

8. The vision is for *social workers practicing in a variety of settings within the health and social services systems*. Some of these settings will be those in which generations of social workers have practiced: hospitals, senior centers, family service agencies, public welfare agencies, Others will be of more recent origins, for example, managed care agencies, employees assistance programs in corporations, newly established community-based hospital clinics and other agencies. In some of these settings, social work will continue to be "the host profession"; in others, the hospital or nursing home, for example, social work will be one of several professions. This vision of the future includes social work as respected members of the staffs of these evolving agencies.

9. The vision of the future includes *social workers participating in and contributing to policy formulation, research, program design, administration, clinical practice, and education for geriatric practice*. The roles are defined as those of the profession in a multi-faceted encompassing fashion, with the necessity for flexibility of role at all system levels.

10. The vision is for *the social work profession to be continually enriched by the knowledge and theories of the behavioral and social sciences, bio-medical disciplines, and the humanities, particularly ethics*. In the vision social workers contribute through research and teaching to the knowledge base of geriatrics from the perspective of their practice and their understanding of older people and the contexts of their lives.

11. This vision requires *improvements in the salaries of geriatric social workers*, so that low salaries are not obstacles in the path of recruitment of students and retention of the highest quality of social workers in the field.

12. The vision *recognizes the creative tensions in the profession*, but the vision for the future, struggles within the profession revolve around over substantive issues, not turf or conflicting idealogies or approaches.

13. The vision is one of *professional education which prepares social workers for competent, effective geriatric practice and develops leaders for future practice* by responsive curricula decisions based on knowledge of changing demographics and emerging needs of client populations.

14. The vision is for *continuous assessments* of changes made in curricula, interdisciplinary team training and faculty accomplishment to maintain high quality in geriatric education.

15. The vision is for *cooperation between Schools of Social Work, Council on Social Work Education, National Association of Social Workers, Associations of State Social Work Licensing* and all other professional associations to initiate and monitor changes to meet these goals to improve the education, training, employment opportunities of geriatric social workers in order to better serve older adults and their families.

RECOMMENDATIONS

Education

Comprehensive Integration of Aging Curricula

1. Standards for the integration of aging curricula into all accredited schools of social work will be established and adopted.

Rationale

Because the majority of social workers will require knowledge of aging in their practice, gerontological content should be incorporated into all social work curricula at both the graduate and undergraduate levels. Association for Gerontology in Higher Education (AGHE), Gerontological Society of America (GSA) and National Association of Social Workers (NASW) have developed core content in social work and aging. Academic and field faculty must be prepared to address this integration into course content related to human growth and development, family practice, diversity as well as direct and community practice methods and health and mental health practicum. Academic and field faculty should work with minority and specialized professional groups to identify content and programs in order to develop curriculum to prepare student for work with diverse elderly populations. Accreditation should include criteria for meeting this standard.

Actions Required

1) Develop consensus standards for content in aging to be part of all social work curricula at BSW and MSW to include criteria for practicum experience.
2) Institutionalize curriculum standards in aging through accreditation process at both the BSW and MSW level.
3) Provide faculty development opportunities in gerontology and geriatrics for social work faculty at both the BSW and MSW level. This includes the dissemination of curriculum models.

Responsible Agents

1) Lead Agency- Council of Social Work Education (CSWE), Social work faculty and deans, AGHE, Association for Gerontology Education in Social Work (AGE-SW);
2) CSWE
3) BHP, universities and colleges, AoA

Expected Outcomes

1) Consensus standards for integrating curricula content in aging will be adopted and incorporated into accreditation standards for schools of social work.
2) Within 2 years one half of the schools of social work will have integrated aging substantially into curricula and within 5 years three quarters of the schools of social work will have accomplished this goal.
3) Within 2 years one half and by 5 years three quarters of the schools of social work will have a core of faculty who have developed the expertise to integrate aging into the curriculum.

Minority Faculty and Student Recruitment

2. Increase the number of minority social work faculty and persons who are recruited, educated, and trained as geriatric social workers.

Rationale

Educators must make substantial modifications in the content of all social work education to include content on minority aging, specific populations, and persons with diseases of stigma. To accomplish this faculty must change their strategic orientations and tactics to develop culturally sensitive and effective interventions for diverse and underserved populations and train their students in the appropriate use of effective intervention strategies. Such efforts should lead to substantial improvement in the quality of services to ethnic minority seniors and greater levels of satisfaction with the services. The Task Force on Minority Issues established by the Gerontological Society of America (GSA) found that there is a tremendous need for new public policy to improve the level of research, funding for education and training of minority health care professionals. Minority faculty recruitment is important for both increasing the effectiveness of education for serving diverse populations and for outreach to minority students.

Action Required

1) Advocate with CSWE, NASW, AGHE and other professional groups serving seniors to adopt the five goals for minority elderly established by the Task Force on Minority Issues of the Gerontology Society of America and to work for the establishment of similar goals for the other undeserved groups included in this report.
2) Work for the establishment of grants, scholarships, and recruitment programs to increase the number of students from ethnic minorities, other life styles and religious groups.

Responsible Agents

GSA Minority Task Force, CSWE, State and National units of the Association of Social Workers.2) NIA, NIMH, BHP, and private foundations.

Expected Outcomes

A significant increase in the number of minority faculty and students and gay and lesbian students in the schools of social work and an increase in the number of these specializing in geriatric social work each year for the next five years.

A Lifespan Matrix for Social Work Education

3. Reorganize curricula in schools of social work on a matrix paradigm which classifies both setting and population and is founded in a life span approach which includes attention to diversity and family and informal support systems.

Rationale

Effective integration of aging content is best accomplished through the rubric of curriculum include both the settings in which social work is practiced and the population from which clients come. Given the number of schools which were identified as not providing a coherent educational program for students interested in geriatric social work, the use of this matrix should improve the quality of geriatric social work education. In addition, the life span approach has the advantage of facilitating the inclusion of content about different cohorts and groups within the older population and their informal support systems, and encourages attention to the variety of settings and systems to which older people come for help. All curricula will be modified to provide sufficient knowledge on culture, communication and techniques of interventions for effective practice with the diverse aged population. The need for social work services should be based on changes in the family system of care and the increasing demands on families.

Actions Required

1) This report will be conveyed officially to CSWE, with the recommendation that CSWE convene a Task Force which shall include appropriate representation from AGE-SW, NASW, and AGHE, and which will be responsible for development of guidelines for curriculum organization. These guidelines are to articulate the recommendation, and are to be disseminated to all schools of social work.

Responsible Agents

CSWE, in collaboration with NASW and AGHE.

Expected Outcomes

Within 2 years the work of the Task Force will have accomplished the development and dissemination of guidelines for the matrix model. Within 5 years at least three quarters of the schools will adopt the guidelines, and will have made substantial curricula changes.

Centers of Excellence in Geriatric Social Work Education and Research

4. Centers of Excellence in Graduate Geriatric Social Work Education and Research will be established to promote leadership in aging and social work.

Rationale

Alzheimer's Research Centers, Cancer Centers, and Geriatric Reach Education Clinical Centers (GRECCs) are model demonstrations of the power of Centers of Excellence in promoting research, adding to knowledge and developing new approaches to practice. Further, Lowy's continuum model of gerontological curriculum development in social work remains a valid model for developing curricula with a higher degree of concentration in aging as well as the broad integration of aging in all social work curricula. Centers for Excellence will be graduate Schools of Social Work with doctoral programs which in addition to the number of aging courses, other criteria should be used to assess gerontology curricula level including: number and stability of students, both academic and field faculty resources and practice sites. Centers of Excellence should have a strong research foundation and an interdisciplinary perspective and work closely with Gerontology Centers, Schools of Medicine and Nursing and allied health programs. Centers for Excellence will be at the forefront of evaluating outcomes of geriatric social work education, training, and practice. Funding for geriatric social work outcomes and intervention research will be sought.

Actions Required

1) Criteria for Centers of Excellence in Graduate Geriatric Social Work Education will be developed and model programs funded as demonstrations.

Responsible Agents

1) AGE-SW, CSWE, BHPr, private foundations,,Schools of Social Work NIH, NIMH, AOA

Expected Outcomes

Within three years 5 schools of social work will be designated and functioning as Centers of Excellence in Geriatric Social Work Education and that number will increase to 10 schools within 5 years.

Social Work Education for Interdisciplinary Team Practice

5. Education for geriatric social work will incorporate didactic and practicum

preparation for work with other disciplines in interdisciplinary practice.

Rationale

Social workers are core members of interdisciplinary teams that serve older clients. The biopsychosocial approach is a major contribution to interdisciplinary decision making. Education should prepare social workers and other health care practitioners for understanding the roles of each discipline and the process for team decision making and care planning in geriatrics. The VA Interdisciplinary Team Training Program (ITTP) and GRECC provide models for interdisciplinary team preparation.

Responsible Agents

Schools and Departments of Social Work in colleges and universities and their training sites would be responsible for collaborating with other disciplines, teaching hospitals and Geriatric Education Centers to sponsor, develop and implement these courses and programs.

Required Action

Cooperative efforts are required to design, develop and implement teaching teams including involvement of hospital and agency personnel. This interdisciplinary education would be documented with letters of agreements between departments and reflected in the curriculum content and agency training arrangements.

Expected Outcomes

Increased number of interdisciplinary teams and more teams designed and developed to deal specifically with the needs of, and services to target populations.

Individual, Organizational, and Policy Level Practice

6. Social work curriculum and practice must address both the micro (service coordination, advocacy and clinical practice) and the macro level (program development, administration and policy in aging).

Rationale

Because of the complexity of geriatric services, there is an increasing need for social workers to coordinate services at a practice, program, and policy level. Social work education with a systems theoretical perspective should prepare social workers for roles of case management, administration, program development and policy level positions as well as direct practice with individuals. Social workers can play a key role in advancing the competency of health professionals in understanding the important role that community service agencies in the community play in meeting health needs. The important role of social workers in case management must be promoted.

Actions Required

1) Standards for social work curricula in aging will include appropriate organization and policy courses as well as direct practice courses including issues of care management;
2) Standards for geriatric case management will be developed and disseminated to promote excellence in practice.

Responsible Agent

1) CSWE and AGE-SW;
2) NASW (Case Management Task Force) including American Society on Aging (ASA) Case Management Task Force Representative

Expected Outcome

1) Within 2 years standards for curricula in aging will be developed and disseminated which include program and policy level practice content
2) Within 2 years a professional standard for social work case management to be developed and disseminated.

Geriatric Social Work Stipends and Fellowships

7. Increase stipend and fellowship support for students interested in careers in geriatric social work.

Rationale

The decline in federal funding of stipends and fellowships, particularly at the MSW level, and the possibility of further cuts makes the recruitment of students for careers in geriatric social work difficult, particularly in the light of the fact that geriatrics is not a field of practice attractive to many social work students. Both private and public funding is needed to increase recruitment of social workers to the field of aging.

Actions Required

An inter-agency task force at the federal level shall be convened, and charged with the responsibility of engaging relevant government officials in the task of securing increased federal funding of stipends and fellowships for social work students, particularly MSW candidates, who are committed to or interested in careers in geriatrics social work. Support within the geriatric traineeship programs will include doctoral and postdoctoral social work positions. These positions will include social work positions in research and as part of interdisciplinary research teams.

Responsible Agents

The Assistant Secretary of DHHS for Aging shall be responsible for convening this task force, and for assigning staff to its work. Required for inclusion on the task force are representatives from VA, HRSA, CMHS, AoA, and NIA, and additional agencies may be invited, at the discretion of the Assistant Secretary, to send representatives to the Task Force. In addition NASW, CSWE, and AGHE will be invited to participate.

Expected Outcomes

Within 3 years: the number of stipends and fellowships offered by agencies of the federal government to MSW candidates interested in or committed to geriatric social work will have increased by 20. Within 5 years: the number of stipends and fellowships provided by the federal government will have increased by 50.

Post Graduate Geriatric Social Work Education

8. Post graduate education and in-service training opportunities for geriatric social workers or social workers in other fields of practice interested in making a career change will be provided.

Rationale

The knowledge base of geriatric social work is a constantly growing and changing one, infused by the findings of researchers in social work and in the social, behavioral, and bio-medical sciences. Geriatric social workers need organized continuing education opportunities in order to maintain and improve their knowledge and skills, and social workers from other fields, (e.g., child welfare,) interested in becoming geriatric social workers require specialized post-graduate education to prepare them for their new practice field. Social work educators must make substantial modification in the content of social work geriatric and gerontology courses to include content on minority elderly, specific populations and aged persons with diseases of stigma.

Action Recommended

The Task Force to be convened by the NASW will assign responsibility for the development of continuing education materials, including guidelines, curriculum outlines, bibliographies, etcetera. The Task Force will also assume responsibility for engaging other relevant organizations and units of the Federal government in furthering the efforts to develop continuing education opportunities, including the provision of funding for such programs.

Responsible Agent

NASW in collaboration with CSWE and AGHE, and from the federal government, HRSA, AoA, and VA.

Expected Outcomes

Within 2 years: the work of the Task Force should be completed, and results disseminated to all schools of social work. The engagement of federal agencies in the work should have been accomplished. Within 5 years: at least half of the schools should be providing opportunities for continuing education in geriatric social work, and there should be increased federal funding provided for post graduate education in geriatric social work.

Evaluation and Continuous Quality Improvement in Practice and Education

9. Continuous Quality Improvement (CQI) strategies are required to responsibly assure the on-going assessment of social work curricula as related to populations served.

Rationale

Improvement in the quality of geriatric social work programs should result in better services to aged clients. The services would be more desired by the clients for increased sensitivity and effective in their ability to meet the needs of elderly persons and persons who care for them. The best way to improve geriatric education and training program is to initiate procedures for continuous quality improvements. Provisions of evaluation using CQI methods, involve consumers, students, and faculty when planning and implementing changes. They also evaluate each change before, during and after they are implemented. Curricula changes must be evaluated and monitored in this fashion. In addition education should prepare practitioners to evaluate their practice and programs for effectiveness in patient outcomes. Social workers should be prepared to utilize data from a variety of sources in order to assess the appropriateness of their interventions. The Pew Foundation reports emphasized the increasing need for all health professionals to be able to utilize technology to manage data and to document accountability.

Action Required

1) Each school of social work will develop a plan to monitor outcomes of curricular changes to address client populations.
2) Social work curriculum will prepare student for intervention research and evaluation of practice.
3) Implementation of a commission or subcommission in accreditation in Council on Social Work Education (CSWE) to have

responsibilities for on-going assessment of relevant curriculum content to insure sound and timely changes in curricula to meet the needs of baccalaureate and master's programs.

Responsible Agents

1, 2) Deans, faculty, students of the various schools and colleges of social work and advisory groups comprised of representative seniors of all of the sub-groups in the community to plan and implement changes in the curricula and the practicum courses of the undergraduate and graduate geriatric social work programs. BHP will disseminate models to increase accountability and effectiveness in geriatric practice.
3) CSWE

Expected Outcomes

Within 5 years each school of social work will develop a plan for monitoring responsiveness to the changing population base for social work services and responding in appropriate curricula. In two years models for intervention research and increased accountability for social work interventions will be developed and disseminated. Within 5 years the majority of social work programs will have adopted these programs.

Employment

Education and Employment

10. Establish standards for education and employment for geriatric social work positions.

Rationale

Social work positions are needed at all levels of geriatric social work practice. BLS and NASW data show that there is a discrepancy between educationally prepared geriatric social workers and persons filling social work positions. There are several important interconnected but distinct issues in the linkage of education and employment for social workers in geriatrics. Social service positions in the aging network have been weak on educational requirements. Social work is a health care which are reimbursed through Medicare and Medicaid payment but must require the appropriate graduate educational requirements and acknowledge social work as a reimbursable service provider for the elderly. Professional organizations in social work frequently develop standards for practice and these must support undergraduate as well as graduate social work levels. NASW has not recruited baccalaureate trained social workers to the organization or to their needs for training or supports. A link between "town and gown" is required to assure that education and training prepares social workers for geriatric practice and that employers require that social work positions are filled with qualified geriatric social workers at the requisite educational level.

Actions Required

1) Standards for geriatric social work force roles to level of training will be developed, clearly articulated and nationally disseminated and subsequently become a requirement for employment in the field.
2) Employers in the field of aging will adopt these standards and designate the a Bachelors in Social Work (BSW) degree for baccalaureate level positions, with supervision/consultation from a Masters in Social Work (MSW), for all undergraduate social work positions in aging. Additionally, employers in geriatric service delivery and specify educational requirements for social work positions at the BSW, MSW, and doctoral levels.

3) Funding from health and social service regulatory agencies will mandate that social work positions be filled by qualified persons with social work education from accredited programs at the specified level.
4) Acknowledging that a graduate degree is the preferred level of education for professional practice, professional organizations will increase outreach to BSW practitioners to include them under professional allegiance.

Responsible Agent

1) Lead agency-National Association of Social Workers (NASW) in collaboration with Council on Social Work Education (CSWE), Association for Gerontology in Higher Education (AGHE), (AGE-SW), Bureau Health Professions (BHP)
2, 3) Area Agency on Aging (AAA) and Health Care Financing Agency (HCFA) (in relation to Medicare and Medicaid certification requirements)
4, 5) NASW and AGE-SW

Expected Outcome

1) Within two years a work group composed of members of the responsible organizations will establish standards and disseminate them.
2, 3) Within five years the standards will be adopted and reflected in regulations and the number of persons holding social work positions in aging without social work education at the appropriate level will decrease according to BLS data and geriatric social workers will be recognized as Medicare and Medicaid providers.
4) NASW and AGE-SW will have significantly increased their BSW representation.

Geriatric Knowledge for Licensure in Social Work

11. All state social work licensing boards for social work licensure examination will include content on their examination of 10% or more of the questions related to working with aged populations.

Rationale

In order to assure that aged populations are receiving adequate and appropriate services, greater efforts must be made to have social workers to demonstrate competency in interventions for older persons. One of the most effective ways of achieving this objective is to have requirements on the content, courses and minimum work experience with aged persons as is done on mental health and child abuse issues.Action Required: Faculty and professional associations will form coalitions and advocacy groups to require the inclusion of content on the elderly populations, including persons of ethnic minority, specific populations and persons with diseases of stigma. Minimum standards will be negotiated between the licensing boards, the legislatures, and the professional groups implement requirements.

Responsible Agents

The responsible parties would NASW working with boards of licensure for social work licenses and state legislatures for passage and implementation of the laws with the minimum requirements with the time lines for implementation.

Expected Outcomes

Within two years guidelines for geriatric content for social work licensure would be developed and disseminated. Within 3 years all state social work licensing boards would have modified their examinations to contain the minimum content required. With 3 years 50% of all states with licensing requirement would have implemented these changes.

Commitment to Public Service

12. Geriatric social work education and practice will emphasize the commitment to public agencies and meeting the needs of underserved populations.

Rationale

The disparity between persons with and without access to appropriate levels of health and social services is increasing. Minority elderly are often more in need of services yet utilize community based care at lower rates than the majority populations. Access issues cut across racial and ethnic groups and also relate to geographic area and most significantly to poverty. Public agencies are most frequently the primary providers of care to underserved populations. NASW reports a decline in social work in public service in contrast to the PEW Foundation increased emphasis on the national need for health professionals in public service and addressing the needs of underserved populations. Declassification or loosing qualifications for social work positions in public agencies has been cited as one major cause of the loss of public service social work positions.

Actions Required

1) Professional organizations will develop statements addressing the declassification issues which have reduced the professional requirements for social work positions.
2) State, county and local governmental agencies will issue policy statements for education requirements for positions with primarily social work tasks and functions.

Responsible Agent

1) NASW, AGE-SW, CSWE
2) State Departments of Aging, Health and Mental Health; County Departments of Public Social Services,Health and Mental Health; and local public agencies.

Expected Outcome

1) Within 2 years standards for the classification of social work positions in public service will be issued and advocated for by professional organizations.
2) Within 5 years, there will be issued increase by 15% the number of social workers in public agencies.

REFERENCES

1. Lowy L. Social work with the aging: The challenge and promise of the later years. New York: Harper & Row, Publishers, 1979, p. 9.
2. National Association of Social Workers. NASW standards for the classification of social work practice (Policy statement 4). Silver Spring, MD: Author, 1981.
3. Shanas E. The family as social support system in old age. The Gerontologist 1979; 19(2): 169–174.
4. Dobrof R, Litwak E. Maintenance of Family Ties of Long-Term Care Patients: Theory and Guide to Practice. Rockville, MD: National Institute of Mental Health, DHEW Publication No. (ADM) 77–400, 1977, pp. 86–110.
5. Butler RN, Lewis M. Aging and Mental Health: Positive Psychosocial and Biomedical Approaches. (Third Edition). St. Louis: The C.V. Mosby Company, 1962, pp. 148–171 and 320–334.
6. Torres-Gil FM. The New Aging: Politics and Change in America. New York: Auburn House, 1992, pp. 9–75, 127–141, and 165–181.
7. U.S. Department of Health and Human Services, Center for Mental Health Services, Report to Congress on Mental Health Clinical Training Program Payback Requirement, June, 1993, p.39.

8. U.S. Department of Health and Human Services, Center for Mental Health Services, Workforce Training and Development for Mental Health Services, February, 1993.
9. Yeo G. Review of current ethnogeriatric curriculum. Working paper series #2. Stanford, CA: Stanford Geriatric Education Center, 1989.
10. Harel Z, McKinney EA, Williams (eds.). Black aged. Newbury Park, CA: Sage, 1990.
11. Minority aging: Essential curricula content for selected health and allied health professions. Health Resources and Services Administration. U.S. Department of Health and Human Services. Washington, D.C.: DHHS Publication No. HRS-P-DV 90-4.
12. Cabot RC. Social service and the art of healing. New York: Moffat, Yard & Co., 1915, pp. 1–192.
13. Tobin SS. The educator as advocate: the gerontologist in an academic setting. Education for Social Work 1973; 9:94–98.
14. Greene R, Barusch A, Connelly R. Social work and gerontology: an update. Final report to the Administration on Aging and Association of Gerontology in Higher Education. Washington, D.C., 1990.
15. U.S. Bureau of Labor Statistics. Current population survey annual average data. Washington, D.C., 1992.
16. Gibelman M, Schervish PH. Who we are: The social work labor force as reflected in the NASW membership. Washington, D.C.: NASW Press, 1994.
17. Peterson DA, Wendt PF. Employment in the field of aging: a survey of professionals in four fields. The Gerontologist 1990; 30(5): 679–85.
18. Lubben LE, Damron-Rodriguez JA, Beck JC. A national survey of aging curriculum in schools of social work. In J. Mellor and R. Solloman, Geriatric social work education. The Haworth Press, Inc., 1992.
19. Lubben JE, Wallace S, Damron-Rodriguez JA, Villa V. Second National Survey of Graduate Social Work Education in Aging. Funded by U.S. Bureau of Health Professions. Unpublished data.
20. Damron-Rodriguez JA, Lubben JE. Multidisciplinary factors in gerontological curriculum adoption in schools of social work. Gerontology and Geriatrics Education 1994; 14(4):39–52.
21. Johnson H, Britton J et al. Foundations for gerontological education. Published as a special issue of the Gerontologist 1980; 20 (3, part II).
22. Nelson G. Personnel and training needs in geriatric social work. Educational Gerontology 1988; 9:307–322.
23. Yeo G. Ethnogeriatric education: need and recommendations. In Shortage of health care professions caring for elderly: recommendations for change. Select Committee on Aging, House of Representatives. Washington, D.C.: Government Printing Office Comm. Pub. #102–915, 1992.
24. Harry L. Minority culture as a factor in communication between doctors and patients. Nevada Public Affairs Review. Reno, NV: Allan Bible Center for Applied Research, University of Nevada, 1994.
25. Kreps GL, Kunimoto EN. Effective communication in multicultural health care settings. Thousand Oaks, CA: Sage Publications, 1994.
25. Yoshikawa TT, Dube WF, Wahby V. Geriatric training in the Department of Veterans Affairs. American Journal of Medicine 1994; 97(Suppl 4A):4A-26S.
26. Moses DG. Correspondence. Washington, D.C.: Social Work Service, Department of Veterans Affairs, 1993.
27. Health professions education for the future: Schools in service to the nation. Pew Health Professions Commission, 1993.

ACKNOWLEDGMENTS

With gratitude, the Study Group acknowledges the help of colleagues in the Federal government.

From the Center for Mental Health Services of Substance Abuse and Mental Health Administration (SAMHSA)
Dr. Paul Wohlford

From the National Institute on Aging
Dr. Ronald Abeles

From the Administration on Aging
Dr. Alfred Duncker
Mr. Bruce Craig

From the Mental Disorders of the Aging Research Branch of the National Institute of Mental Health (NIMH)
Dr. Barry Lebowitz

From the Department of Veterans Affairs
Jan Feazeld

4

Long-Term Care

Margaret Dimond, Donna Lind Infeld, Alice Kethley, and Eric Pfeiffer

THE STATE OF THE ART OF GERIATRIC LONG-TERM CARE EDUCATION AND TRAINING

Introduction

Defining Geriatric Education and Training for the Continuum of Long-Term Care Services

The purpose of this chapter is to focus on the need for geriatric education and training for a wide range of health professionals and paraprofessionals who provide care to elderly persons in order to meet the future demand for quality long-term care services. There is substantial overlap between geriatrics and long-term care, but the two terms are not synonymous. Geriatrics is a medical and health care specialty which is practiced in most long-term care settings, but long-term care involves more than the practice of geriatric medicine. It is a broader concept, incorporating quality of life, environmental appropriateness, family involvement, and other aspects of daily living. While geriatric education focuses on diseases of aging, this discussion takes a broader perspective, addressing care needed as a result of a range of functional and other changes related to aging.

Long-term care includes a range of services that addresses the health, personal care, and social needs of individuals who lack some capacity for self care. Services may be continuous or intermittent but are delivered for a sustained period to individuals who have a demonstrated need, usually measured by some index of functional dependency.[1] It is critical that long-term care be viewed as a perspective, not as a specific location of care provision. While long-term care includes services provided in a full range of settings, from an individual's home to a nursing facility, this chapter does not address training for informal care providers. Further, while long-term care generally addresses the needs of a range of patient populations, for the purpose of this discussion, the focus is on care of the elderly.

Long-term care is sometimes used synonymously with chronic care. Medicare eligible individuals who become users of long-term care services suffer from diseases which are chronic, such as Alzheimer's, arthritis, diabetes, congestive heart failure, depression, and chronic obstructive pulmonary disease. Such diseases require health care over many years in a variety of settings (home, clinics, nursing homes, etc.) and a workforce which is trained in gerontology and geriatrics. Long-term care can also result from life-long disabilities such as mental retardation and other developmental disabilities.

Multidisciplinary and interdisciplinary are two additional terms which are critical to this discussion and often cause confusion. In a recent paper, Clark presents clear definitions of these terms. Multidisciplinary "may be defined as bringing various disciplines together to understand a particular problem or experience, such as the process of ageing."[2] Interdisciplinary or interprofessional refers to "the level at which real integration of perspectives occurs. Instead of parallel lines of communication among different disciplines, intersecting lines of communication and collaboration are the norm. Integration and modification of the contributions of different disciplines take place in the light of input from other professions."[2]

It also is important to understand the distinction between geriatrics and gerontology. Geriatrics refers to the clinical practice by physicians and other health care professionals involved with treating elderly patients. On the other hand, gerontology is the interdisciplinary study of older persons, including disciplines such as economics, psychology, sociology, political science, and many other academic and applied fields. It is critical that health care providers, both professionals and paraprofessionals, understand both geriatric care and gerontology. That is, in addition to knowing about the diseases and conditions being treated, they also need to know about older people as people and as patients. They need to know how to effectively communicate with older people, how to be supportive and respond to their complex array of concerns and problems. It is important to note that even health care professionals who have received specialty training in geriatrics do not necessarily receive systematic coverage of the long-term care perspective. Even some health care providers in geriatrics who see themselves as specialists, may not have been exposed to the complete range of long-term care settings.

Another term which often causes confusion is allied health. One useful definition of allied health is "a large cluster of health care related professions and personnel whose functions include assisting, facilitating, or complementing the work of physicians and other specialists in the health care system, and who choose to be identified as allied health personnel.[3] Because there is no widely accepted definition, for purposes of this discussion, the above definition will be used but modified to include those who meet the first part of the definition, whether or not they choose to be identified as allied health personnel.

Populations of Concern

The population of concern tends to suffer from a wide range of physical and/or mental disabilities, most of which are chronic in nature, some having evolved from life-long developmental diseases and disabilities. Whatever their etiology, many persons spend much of their older years facing serious limitations caused by changes in health or functional status.

The increasing need for long-term care geriatric education and training is being driven by the changing demographic face of

America. Most geriatric educators and practitioners, health care planners, and legislators know the statistics underlying the growth of the aging population. As identified in the Introduction of the book, there will be a large population of older adults living with chronic disabilities and residing in the community. Education and training for future geriatric and long-term care health professionals should be based on the projected demographics and health care needs of this aging population.

Education and training for long-term care is essential for a broad range of health care providers including: physicians, dentists, pharmacists, podiatrists, nurse practitioners and physician assistants, registered and licensed practical nurses, therapists (physical, occupational, speech, music and activities), nutritionists and dietitians, nursing aides, homemakers, chore workers, and companions, social workers and other providers of mental health services (including psychiatric nurses, psychologists, etc.), administrators and managers, case managers, discharge planners, informal caregivers (including drivers of vehicles transporting elderly to and from services), and volunteers. This list is not exhaustive; it simply suggests the extent of disciplines and fields needing further education and training. Education needs to encompass both didactic and clinical training in a broad array of geriatrics and gerontological areas identified in the recommendations of this chapter.

State of the Art: Past

First Generation Education and Training Programs

Attracting professionals and paraprofessionals to work with this growing population has been historically difficult partially because their illnesses are long-term, with little gratification from progress or cure. The difficulty has been exacerbated by lack of funding to lure faculty and students into this area of health care. Financial support for interdisciplinary and/or single discipline training programs has been sporadic over the years and has come from both the private and the public sectors. University-based interdisciplinary training programs got their first big boost with the passage of the Older Americans Act in 1965. Under Title V of that landmark legislation, monies were available for student stipends and faculty retraining in gerontology as well as administrative costs to support the academic interdisciplinary structure. During the same period private monies established major centers, such as the Ethel Percy Andrus Gerontology Center at the University of Southern California. Professionals from around the nation were attracted with stipends supported by grants for academic programs and summer short courses. Funds were made available from the National Institute of Mental Health and the Administration on Aging for these programs. Though these early centers did not focus on long-term care, they trained a workforce of researchers, educators, and practitioners who became the catalyst and backbone of gerontological and geriatric education.

Veterans Administration

Within the Veterans Administration (VA) the concept of Geriatric Research, Education, and Clinical Centers (GRECCs) was developed in 1973. Between 1975 and 1980, eight GRECCs were established. In 1980, a total of 15 GRECCs were authorized. All GRECCs are located in VA medical centers affiliated with colleges of medicine. GRECCs have been the cornerstone of a number of major geriatric programs in health science centers across the country. The majority of GRECCs have had a topical focus which commonly include disease or problem areas central to long-term care, to wit: health services research; diabetes mellitus; cognitive disorders; sexual dysfunction; bone disease; nutrition; and other studies including attention to pharmacological issues in older patients.

All of the GRECCs, by definition, have a formal educational component. In a number of VA facilities with GRECCs, a formal fellowship in geriatrics has been added, thereby enhancing the educational component of the GRECCs. What is particularly important about the VA GRECC program is, that unlike other programs such as the AOA Long-Term Care Gerontology Centers Program, it is a continuing program, providing a nidus of geriatric and long-term educational activity, at least in selected areas of the country.

Administration on Aging Long-Term Care Gerontology Centers

In 1980, the Administration on Aging (AOA) in the Department of Health and Human Services (DHHS) began a program of university-based Long-Term Care (LTC) Gerontology Centers to address national long-term care issues.[4] Initially, five such centers were established in university settings which already had a significant commitment to geriatrics. The program eventually grew to ten centers nationally, with the added dimension to serve as regional Resource Centers on Long-Term Care (for the HHS regions, I-X). Unlike the VA GRECCs, these LTC Gerontology Centers were never placed on a continuing funding basis. Thus the impact they had on the field was variable; some centers survived under alternative funding sources; others became dormant, while still others disappeared altogether. No formal evaluation of the AOA Long-Term Care Gerontology Centers was ever undertaken. Yet it is clear that they developed interest, expertise, and a focus on long-term care in many universities and medical schools.

Two somewhat casual attitudes toward these center programs prevailed. One of these opined that the mere availability of LTC Gerontology Center grant funds would stimulate interest in long-term care in many additional health sciences centers, even those not receiving funds. Another opinion held that evaluation of the centers program or of individual centers was not needed. If a center survived beyond initial funding, that center was successful; if not, not. These opinions have to be taken with a large grain of salt, since the reasons for ending the program were primarily political (changes of administration nationally and within AOA) rather than the fact that the long-term care problem had been solved. Interestingly, the current AOA administration has again made long-term care an area of priority initiatives, funding several special long-term care resource centers and other projects emphasizing home and community-based services, but not necessarily education or training.

Bureau of Health Professions' Geriatric Education Centers

In 1983, the Bureau of Health Professions of the Health Resources and Services Administration, established Geriatric Education Centers. These Centers target a broad student audience including professionals working in all health care settings, with a strong focus on faculty development.

While some who receive training at GECs will practice in long-term care settings, there is no specific focus on long-term care in these Centers and no way to identify trainees or other participants who work in long-term care. From their inception, the number of federally funded GECs grew to a high of 38 in 1989.[6] However, by 1994 that number had declined to 20 and the amount of future funding is unknown. Awards over the past twelve years totalled $83.3 million in funding, with the most recent year's funding at $6.3 million. Data is available on enrollees (trainees with 40 or more hours of training), participants (trainees with less than 40 hours of training) and all trainees (who received any training) in GEC programs. Table 4.1 displays the numbers of each type of trainee. In total, over 225,000 persons, representing over 26 professions, were reached by some level of GEC training between 1984 and 1993. Table 4.2 presents the distribution of their disciplines. Nursing, medicine, and social work are clearly the most frequently represented professions in GEC training programs, accounting for 53.0 percent of participants and 66.2 percent of enrollees during ten years of program operation. Two specific areas in which GECs have had particular impact have been in ethnogeriatrics and elder abuse.[6] As GECs are known for areas of expertise, long-term care would be an appropriate area of expertise for additional GECs because, despite their foci on geriatrics, none, to date, has emphasized this critical topic.

While funding over the years from these various federal sources has been limited, it has had a significant impact on those it reached. There is better understanding in the professions of what various health providers need to know, (eg., geriatrics education) and better education and training for long-term care provision is available. Federal funding helped build a leadership cadre which is still active and influential in the field. Limited funds have had a substantial impact. Unfortunately, as funds dry up, education and training centers often do not continue interdisciplinary training in gerontology and long-term care. This is often due to the organizational structures of most universities where interdisciplinary programs require additional time and resources for organizing activities across disciplinary boundaries. Faculty and staff are typically paid for work within a specific department and time required to do work beyond that department must be supported by external funds.

Robert Wood Johnson Foundation Teaching Nursing Homes

At about the same time as the establishment of GECs, in 1982 the Robert Wood Johnson Foundation (RWJF) launched its Teaching Nursing Home (TNH) initiative. Eleven academic schools of nursing were funded to work in collaboration with a skilled nursing facility to improve nursing care. The purpose of the RWJF-TNH Program was to entice faculty and students from schools of nursing to learn about long-term care for older adults and to practice together in nursing homes affiliated with these eleven schools of nursing.[7] Although some participating schools of nursing included a research component in their program objectives, the majority of the schools focused on education and practice, including interdisciplinary practice. Continuation of the programs beyond the funding stage was problematic for all sites. However, the initiative raised an awareness of the potential for enhanced education and training for health professionals in long-term care through collaborative efforts between academic and long-term-care sites.

Table 4.1 Number of GEC Trainees by Year and Type of Trainee, Fiscal Year 1984–1993[6]

FY	Participants	Enrollees	Trainees
1984	953	36	989
1985	964	44	1,008
1986	7,250	575	7,825
1987	12,333	1,042	13,375
1988	24,098	1,222	25,320
1989	31,985	1,813	33,798
1990	48,193	1,755	49,948
1991	33,688	11,674	45,362
1992	19,250	8,327	27,577
1993	16,449	3,784	20,233
TOTAL	**195,163**	**30,272**	**225,435**

Participants = Individuals with less than 40 hours training;
Enrollees = Individuals with 40+ hours training;
Trainees = Participants + Enrollees.

National Institute on Aging Teaching Nursing Homes

During the same period, the National Institute on Aging (NIA) launched its own teaching nursing home programs through academic medical schools. These programs trained medical students in geriatrics as well as providing research support. Medical students in programs received didactic and clinical training, following geriatric patients in nursing homes and the patients' own homes. The Teaching Nursing Homes were important initiatives that continue to have impact in several locations. However, neither the RWJ or the NIA initiative lasted long enough to institutionalize such vital training as part of university education.

John A. Hartford Foundation

The other major player among foundations has been the John A. Hartford Foundation. Since 1985, the Hartford Foundation has conducted a major grant program in the area of geriatric education, focusing on faculty development and on academic geriatrics recruitment, through grants to universities with strength in geriatric medicine. In 1994, Hartford has awarded two grants to the American Geriatrics Society, for enhancement of training in geriatrics in various nonmedical specialties, and in subspecialties of internal medicine. Still more recently, Hartford has expressed a specific interest in interdisciplinary education in geriatrics. While none of these programs have dealt specifically with long-term care, the recently expressed interest on interdisciplinary training in geriatrics comes closest to addressing long-term care including a interdisciplinary approach.

Summary

It should be noted that within the National Institutes of Health, NIA and the National Institute of Mental Health (NIMH) both have activities related to aging. However, in most cases their initiatives focus on research rather than education or training.

All of the gerontological and geriatric training programs of the past 30 years have contributed to the beginning of the body of knowledge available today. However, weaknesses include a lack of secure and ongoing funding and the absence of a commitment by the federal government to designate an agency with permanent responsibility and funds to address the workforce needs for provision of long-term care services. Funding for such programs has moved from one federal agency to another, each having fixed resources for limited years. Nationally, training of professionals in long-term care has been approached as though the need were short term. In practice, the need for a trained workforce to provide care to chronically physically and mentally ill older adults is long-term and growing.

State of the Art: Present

Current State of Geriatric Long-Term Care Education and Training

Too few health professionals are being prepared to meet the long-term health care needs of the aging population. This conclusion is repeated in nearly all studies and surveys of educational programs which prepare health care professionals. Numerous reports address the significant current and emerging issues around the preparation of health professionals for a reformed health care system. Few address the problems specific to the preparation of health care providers to deliver quality long-term care for aging adults in a new system, and virtually none address education and training issues around the delivery of quality long-term care for older adults. Butler[5] refers to a "geriatric imperative," driven by the demographics of an aging society, increased chronic illness and health care costs which should, but has not, sufficiently affected the focus of education and training programs for geriatric health care professionals.

The Bureau of Health Professions (BHPr) of the Health Resources and Services Administration (HRSA), whose responsibility it is to improve the education and quality of the nation's supply of health care professionals, has repeatedly pointed out the deficiencies in the supply of health care providers for the elderly. Among the issues noted in various reports are a general shortage of personnel prepared to care for the elderly; specific shortages of allied health professionals and nurses; shortage of primary care providers; and problems associated with the delivery of services in rural areas. Other areas of concern noted by the BHPr are the lack of faculty with geriatric preparation to serve as role models in practice and research, the need for interdisciplinary educational preparation in geriatrics, and the need to enhance curricular content in chronic illness and long-term care.[9, 10] In reports to the President and Congress, HRSA has pointed out the negative impact on geriatric education of limited qualified faculty, inadequate and uncertain funding for geriatric education, and underemphasis on health promotion, disease prevention, and long-term care.[9, 10]

A brief overview of the education and training of key health professionals for the care of older adults shows that the general issues reported by the BHPr are restated in documents pertaining to specific health disciplines, i.e. medicine, nursing, dentistry, allied health, and health administration. The focus of concern in these reports is an over-

Table 4.2 Number and Percent of Participants and Enrollees, by Discipline, 1984–1993[6]

Discipline	Number of Participants	Percent of Participants	Number of Enrollees	Percent of Enrollees
Nursing	49,513	25.4%	7,482	24.7%
Allopathic/Osteopathic Medicine	31,756	16.3%	6,110	20.2%
Social Work	21,933	11.3%	6,441	21.3%
Dentistry	7,787	4.0%	888	2.9%
Health Administration	6,485	3.3%	1,694	5.6%
Pharmacy	6,187	3.2%	967	3.2%
Occupational Therapy	4,311	2.2%	451	1.5%
Psychology	4,207	2.2%	650	2.1%
Health Education	2,956	1.5%	265	0.9%
Dietetics	1,902	1.0%	308	1.0%
Physical Therapy	2,804	1.4%	743	2.5%
Gerontology	2,322	1.2%	607	2.0%
Public Health	1,550	0.8%	579	1.9%
Counseling	1,322	0.7%	135	0.4%
Speech Pathology	950	0.5%	94	0.3%
Dental Hygiene	1,352	0.7%	192	0.6%
Physician Assistants	897	0.5%	140	0.5%
Optometry	987	0.5%	67	0.2%
Nutrition	623	0.3%	75	0.2%
Sociology	568	0.3%	194	0.6%
Recreational Therapy	513	0.3%	59	0.2%
Respiratory Therapy	439	0.2%	29	0.1%
Audiology	364	0.2%	87	0.3%
Podiatry	240	0.1%	59	0.2%
Home Economics	78	0.0%	28	0.1%
Art Therapy	68	0.0%	32	0.1%
Unidentified	43,049	21.1%	1,896	6.3%
TOTAL	**195,163**	**100.0%**	**30,272**	**100.0%**

Participants = Individuals with less than 40 hours training. Enrollees = Individuals with 40+ hours training.

all deficiency in the education and training of health professionals in geriatrics. Given these inadequacies, it is not surprising to find that very limited attention has been paid to the unmet need for health professionals with specific expertise in long-term care of older adults.

Faculty Shortages

A recurrent theme throughout published reports is the desperate need to increase the numbers of geriatric faculty, particularly minority faculty, to serve as academic and clinical role models. In spite of limited funding for geriatric fellowships for faculty training in geriatric medicine and dentistry, inadequate numbers of faculty with knowledge and skills in geriatrics are being prepared. Reasons for this state of affairs are somewhat different depending on the discipline, but in general can be traced to lack of interest in primary care, especially primary care geriatrics, absence of incentives or funding for current faculty to refocus their practice and scholarship on geriatrics, and considerably less pay for some primary care providers in geriatrics when compared with specialists. It is not uncommon, in disciplines other than medicine, to find that faculty are predominantly prepared at the masters level, are not full-time faculty, and yet have major responsibility for the teaching or clinical supervision of students in settings whose clients are primarily older adults.[8, 10] In one survey, forty percent of the total nursing faculty (graduate and undergraduate), had no specific preparation in gerontology or geriatrics, and 77 percent of the reporting schools indicated that clinical preceptors for students learning to care for older adults were not prepared in gerontology.[8]

Geriatrics Curriculum

Closely linked with the lack of an adequate number of geriatric faculty in educational institutions is insufficient curricular emphasis on geriatrics. In some health disciplines it is necessary to distinguish between geriatric curricula for undergraduate and graduate study. For example, in a 1987 survey of 498 baccalaureate programs by the American Nurses Association,[10, 12] it was apparent that geriatric content was most likely to be integrated throughout the curriculum rather than covered in specific required geriatric courses. At the masters level, programs which prepare geriatric nurse practitioners include required courses with specialized content in geriatrics. It is generally the case that programs which prepare family or adult nurse practitioners rely more heavily on the integration of geriatric content rather than specific courses in geriatric care. Besdine[13] argues for a distinction between undergraduate and graduate curricular strategies for medicine, as well as pharmacy, nursing, and allied health education.

In the field of health care administration, little emphasis is placed on long-term care in the overall curriculum.[11] Most faculty have limited long-term care background or experience, so core courses which are supposed to address all health care settings tend to give little attention to nursing facilities or home and community-based services. Specific skills and knowledge needed to manage senior housing, assisted living, retirement communities, skilled nursing facilities, home care, and adult day care is rarely provided. A growing number of graduate and undergraduate Association of University of Health Administration (AUPHA) member programs have begun offering electives in long-term care administration, but most often this entails one elective course, taken by few students, and trying to address the full range of facility and community-based services for the elderly. From 1986–89, with funds from the Robert Wood Johnson Foundation, AUPHA conducted a Long-Term Care Administration Education program which included supporting ten faculty members to spend a semester in a long-term care program or facility. These faculty have increased the presence of long-term care in their respective programs, but much more is needed.

Another problem in the development of high quality long-term care administrators is created by licensure requirements which act as barriers to career access. State nursing home administrator licensure requirements, designed to improve quality of care, make it difficult for administrators to move between states and even more difficult for administrators from other health care sectors to move into nursing home management. To the extent that nursing homes are part of the long-term care continuum, it is dysfunctional to separate them out for different administrator requirements.

Interdisciplinary Education and Training

Given the general failure, to date, to develop and demand required discipline-specific curricula in geriatrics for students in the health professions, it is understandable, though not acceptable, that interdisciplinary curricula in geriatrics has not taken root in health professions schools. Interdisciplinary care is necessary to meet the complex health problems of older adults.[5] One discipline cannot meet all the health care needs of this population. The philosophy of team care is built on the assumption that the highest quality of care is provided by a team of experts in geriatric care. The Interdisciplinary Team Training Program (ITTP) offered in selected VAMCs across the country is an example of a program which prepares physicians, nurses, psychologists, social workers, pharmacists, and occupational and physical therapists to collaborate in the care of older adults.[14]

Except for the relatively few programs, such as the ITTP, the struggle to overcome barriers to interdisciplinary education continue. Some of the barriers can be identified as territoriality, others have to do with crowded discipline-specific curricula which leave little time for interdisciplinary courses or practica, noncomparable levels of students across disciplines, various levels of qualified faculty across disciplines, required versus elective courses, differing values toward geriatric content across disciplines, and differing values with regard to interdisciplinary student experiences by clinical practice settings. Older adult issues are often complex and not well addressed by a single disciplinary perspective. Therefore, an interdisciplinary approach to care is critical. Skills at working within a team environment do not happen on their own; they must be taught and developed.

Clinical Practice Sites

Despite the fact that the majority of older adults live in and receive health care in the home or community-based settings, and most of the illnesses of old age are chronic and long-term, clinical practice sites for student experiences continue to focus primarily on the acute hospital. A survey of schools of nursing indicated that hospitals ranked first as an undergraduate clinical practice site for care of older adults, followed closely by nursing homes or extended care facilities.[8] To prepare for the real world of long-term care clinical practice sites used in geriatric long-term care educational programs should be focused in home and community-based clinical settings. At the same time, some exposure to practice in acute settings and long-term care institutions should be a component of every health professions student's clinical experience. A full range of practica sites will prepare students with the necessary skills and knowledge to provide quality continuum of care which will accommodate the many transitions within the health care delivery system experienced by older adults.

One example of the new focus on treating elderly patients through the various transitions of their care is the development of The National Chronic Care Consortium (NCCC). Established in 1991, NCCC is a voluntary network of 24 non-profit health provider groups located in sixteen states. These provider networks are dedicated to transforming and improving the delivery of services to people with serious and persistent chronic conditions. NCCC is working to reform the delivery system by serving as a national laboratory for developing and refining strategies and techniques for integrating care, financing, information systems, and system management across time, place, and profession. While the NCCC is trying to lead the way toward an integrated acute and long-term care health system, its focus is solely on demonstration and delivery, not on training or education of personnel to work in this new, evolving system. In addition to NCCC, other developments in health care delivery, including the growth of managed care arrangements, may lead to hiring based on team skills. However, at the present time, despite the need for team delivered services, hiring rarely focusing on the team approach.

Rural Geriatric Care

NCCC organizations and their efforts to integrate acute and long-term care are concentrated in urban areas. In this, and many other ways, rural areas have even greater deficiencies in geriatric care. Geriatric health care in rural areas is increasingly critical. According to the 1990 census, 25 percent of all older people in the United States (7.7 million older Americans) live in rural areas. Although the delivery of health care is a general concern for rural-dwelling populations, shortages of health care providers in rural areas has a disproportionate impact on the elderly. Rural areas have a higher concentration of elderly and higher rates of chronic illness and disability. There is a shortage of the full spectrum of health care providers in rural America including physicians, social workers, dentists, nurses, physical therapists, psychologists, lab technicians, x-ray technicians, and pharmacists.[15] Nurses and social workers are a critical component of the rural health care delivery system. In particular, geriatric nurse practitioners are prepared to manage common acute and chronic health problems of older adults and are more likely to practice in rural settings than physicians. Importantly, nurse practitioners are reimbursed by Medicare for care delivered in long-term care settings in non-metropolitan communities.[16]

Multiskilled Workers

Given the general shortage of health care providers, closures of small rural hospitals, and reduced services such as transportation, the need for "multiskilled" health care workers is increasing. One potential major resource for multiskilled workers is among allied health professionals. The future of such professionals may depend on the ability to envision and develop educational programs that prepare individuals to provide services in more than one arena. Leaders among allied health professionals are being urged by such prestigious groups as the Pew Foundation to consider different, even radically different, educational programs which would prepare professionals for multiskilled jobs in medically underserved and rural communities. Multiskilled workers are necessary and especially appropriate in long-term care settings. Many long-term care jobs with overlapping responsibilities create natural multiskilled opportunities. For example, patient assessments could be conducted by nurses, social workers, or other health care professionals. In addition, positions in which a narrow range of skills are used can be combined with other related job tasks. For example, therapists who are specialists in one function could develop skills in other therapies.

Student Recruitment and Development

Recruitment and development of geriatric health care students, particularly students from minority and underrepresented geographic areas, is also a serious concern. This is especially so given the evidence that underrepresented minority health profession graduates are more likely to enter primary care and to voluntarily practice in or near primary care health workforce shortage areas.[17] Several related factors may account for the dearth of students in geriatric majors. Among these are the low status of working with the elderly, lower compensation, perceived unpleasantness of working with the elderly, and lack of interest in or knowledge of long-term care.[7] In addition, other contributing factors are lack of geriatric faculty, particularly faculty of color, to serve as role models and mentors; the relatively small pool of minority applicants to health professional schools from whom to select and admit qualified students; the difficulty for rural-dwelling individuals to relocate to urban settings to attend school; the generally ineffective career ladder programs for advancing in the health professions, and the emphasis on urban care settings for student clinical practica. A major factor in the dearth of student applicants is the lack of financial support for these students. Financial incentives may be the most attractive motivator for the recruitment and retention of health professional students preparing for a career in long-term care for older adults.

Non-licensed Providers

Although much of the informal care of chronically ill and frail older adults is provided by family members, formal programs of care depend extensively on non-licensed providers. Home health aides and nursing home aides are responsible for the daily care of homebound and institutionalized elders. Many nursing home aides have had little or no formal training. In 1986 only 17 states had mandated training requirements for nursing home aides, and there were no federal standards for training.[19] With the passage of the Nursing Home Reform Act of 1987 (P.L. 100-203), nursing aides are now required to receive a minimum of 75 hours of state-approved training and must pass a competency examination to become certified. Facilities are also charged with providing continuing education opportunities. While these regulations are a significant improvement, there remains a lack of identification and endorsement of minimum standards of education and training for all nursing home aides, and there is no data to identify the most effective way to educate individuals with minimal educational background, poor reading and writing skills, and minimal English-speaking skills.

Outside of nursing homes, care for homebound older adults is provided by a wide array of non-licensed providers, including home health aides, chore workers, personal care aides, and homemakers. There is much less standardization of educational requirements for these workers than there is for nursing home aides. In a recent survey, at least 12 different titles were commonly used in 50 states for these workers; and training requirements ranged from 40–120 hours.[18, 20] As with caregivers in nursing homes, many home health aides have minimal education, do not speak English, and have poor reading and writing skills. Of particular concern among home care workers is the fact that they often work alone, with little or no direct supervision. Both nursing home and home care aides are poorly paid and have high turnover rates. Conflicts between the elderly clients and aides have been documented,[16, 20] and both physical and psychological abuse are potential threats.[22] The need for quality education and training of non-licensed caregivers, and supervision and encouragement from health professionals (nurses, social workers, and health care administrators) is critical if older adults are to receive the quality of care they deserve.

State of the Art: Future

Vision of Long-Term-Care Services

In order to explore the future system of education and training for long-term care providers, it is first necessary to visualize the future system of long-term care service delivery. The goal should be to assure future long-term care with a very different model than long-term care of today. This model will be based on a humane and dignified system of services, responsive to the changing service needs of the individuals whose capacity for self-care has been reduced by chronic, physical, and/or mental disorders. The goal of this system will be to keep people in their homes as long as possible, and when that is not possible, then to assure their care in the most appropriate setting. The system will be designed to promote maximum functional independence and quality of life, with kindness and dignity. This long-term care system will seamlessly include preventive, restorative, rehabilitative, supportive, and end-of-life services, in a variety of home, community, and residential care settings. Long-term care is part of overall health and well being and should be integrated within managed care efforts, prevention strategies, and primary care delivery. Unfortunately, this is a very different system than the current set of fragmented services, lacking common funding, shared information, and effective coordinating mechanisms.

One of the key changes in the future long-term care system will be its ability to regularly interact with, and not be viewed as separate form, the nation's acute health care system. Funding for "episodes of illness" will include acute and long-term phases of that illness. As a result, hospitals, nursing homes, and home care settings will all consistently be viewed as part of the geriatric care system. As a result, care of the chronically ill and disabled will assume an importance equal to the provision of acute health care services in the personal and national value system.

This vision is consistent with the mission of the National Chronic Care Consortium (NCCC). As described in its strategic plan, the basis of that future is Geriatric Care Networks (GCNs) which will contain:

1. an integrated continuum of prevention, acute care, transitional care and long-term care (community and residential) services, with providers following a common set of care protocols and quality measures;
2. self-help assistance that empowers disabled adults and their family caregivers to optimize functional independence and well-being;
3. specialized short-term care services under a common auspice or strategic alliance including: (a) geriatric assessment and consultation, (b) inpatient transitional care, (c) geriatric rehabilitation, (d) adult day health (rehabilitation oriented), (e) home health/home help services (rehabilitation orientation), (f) caregiver support, and (g) self-help technology in chronic care;
4. patient/client access to the complete spectrum of chronic care services from any point they contact the care network;
5. centralized care management (coordinated with primary care physicians) with responsibilities across the spectrum of acute and long-term-care services as needed by clients in order to maintain continuity of care throughout the life cycle of a given chronic condition or set of conditions;
6. specialized organizational capability in chronic care: a) strategic planning, b) financial management, c) information management, d) in-service training and education, e) research and development, f) marketing management, g) quality, and h) health direction;
7. provider-based managed care capability for heavy use, chronic care clients, including arrangements with third-party payers using a capitated, outcome-oriented, episode-based approach covering both acute and long-term care services.[21]

Vision of Long-Term Care Education and Training

Future professionals will be trained in the entire range of long-term care problems. Training will include experiences in home, residential, community, and hospital settings. Interdisciplinary settings will be the sites for training, with each trainee incorporating an interdisciplinary approach to long-term care problems. This may include multi-skilled professionals and/or cross-training. Professionals will be trained and competent to appreciate and respond to individual cultural and spiritual differences, regardless of their own cultural background.

Geriatric education and training programs will be available to prepare health and social service professionals and caregivers to provide skilled and sensitive care for all aspects of the long-term care experience. This experience is a developmental process including psychological, social, economic, and other components and incorporating didactic as well as clinical content.

In order to meet this mandate, a comprehensive long-term care curriculum should be an integral part of the education of a wide range of professions. The following section outlines a core of knowledge and skills for all professional and paraprofessional providers as well as non-core areas targeted to specific provider groups. These knowledge and skill areas are essential for provision of quality long-term-care services in the future.

Core Knowledge and Skill Areas for Long-Term-Care Provision. All professionals and paraprofessionals need knowledge of basic gerontology/geriatrics, team practice, cultural sensitivity/competency, family/informal caregiver dynamics and mental health issues (depression, alcohol abuse, drug abuse, risk identification), how to prevent client dependency, and respect for individual differences (spiritual/ethical values). Health promotion and disease prevention are also needed areas. Knowledge of preventing hospitalization and improving hospital stays for elderly patients should be a central component of education for all long-term care providers.

Direct service staff, especially, need to learn techniques to assure their own personal safety, prevent burnout, build supportive networks, as well as developing understanding of documentation and record keeping, laws, regulations, policy issues, and reimbursement.

In addition to the core content and skills described above, professionals need to know about the full array of community resources and possess strong supervisory skills.

All of these core areas and skills need to be part of basic career/job preparation for future employees in long-term care. Because many current providers did not gain these knowledge areas in their professional training, they may need to be covered in a continuing education/ training format for those already in the field.

Site-Specific Knowledge and Skill Areas for Long-Term-Care Provision. In addition to these general content and skill areas, various providers providing care in specific settings need more targeted training and/or education. These include:

Home Care

- Physicians need medical management skills with team training in interdisciplinary care planning and case review, communication, and working with a team;
- Incentives are needed for Nurse Practitioners and Physician Assistants to work in home care environments;
- Registered nurses need improved knowledge of geriatric patient assessment, in-home assessment (environment), and medication issues specific to older adults;
- Social workers need a better understanding of the medical context of geriatric care including skills in observation of physiological effects of prescription medications. Social workers also need knowledge of geriatric mental health because they often carry the core of mental health responsibility for the team;
- LPNs should be used, when appropriate, with supervision, as part of the team in home care settings;
- Therapists need to appreciate the potential for rehabilitation of older patients, how to increase motivation using benchmarks for older people, environmental adaptation, and realistic timeframe expectations;
- Case Managers should be trained to help avoid hospitalization. They need the ability to draw on additional team members including clergy, financial advisors, and dietitians and nutritionists who should all be part of the assessment and care planning process;
- Nursing Aides need better communication skills for working with older patients and for communicating with team members. Observation skills also need development.

Community-based Care

(such as Adult Day Care, Day Respite,

On Lok/PACE)
Many of the skills identified above also apply to community-based care provision. In addition, the following are particular to these sites.

- Drivers who transport Alzheimer's disease patients need special training on communication and patient management;
- Managers need expanded skills in recruiting and training volunteers. They also need to understand motivation, group process, fund raising, and grant writing more than in non-long-term care environments.

Housing-based Settings
(such as Naturally Occurring Retirement Communities, Retirement Housing, HUD Housing, Assisted Living, Board and Care Homes)

- Managers need to understand regulations related to the health care environment and appropriate provision of care in each setting. They need to be aware of the full continuum of care including Area Agencies on Aging. Managers should potentially hire additional staff (social work, nursing, case managers, activities therapists) to meet resident needs. At a minimum, managers should be able to facilitate use of homemakers/chore, companions, and other home workers;
- In Assisted Living, aides and caregivers need to understand when a setting is no longer able to meet patient needs, both legally and in terms of best placement for care.

The future system of long-term care services and training must develop and expand dramatically and incorporate continuing quality improvement efforts, as it develops, to meet predictable future levels of need for care. This future will not occur by itself. Significant initiatives, described in the Recommendations which follow, are needed to shape this future. As demand for services continues to grow, training of personnel for such a system must gain national priority, with programs implemented at national, state, and community levels. If this development does not occur, a significant crisis of long-term care delivery will develop. In order to achieve the vision of a humane and dignified long-term care system, responsive to the changing needs of individuals with chronic disabilities, the following recommendations are put forward.

RECOMMENDATIONS

Funding for Long-Term-Care Education and Training

1. There should be on-going federal funding for long-term-care education and training for professionals and paraprofessionals working within the long-term care system.

Rationale
The demographic and health care needs of a rapidly aging population have accelerated the need for education and training in home, community-based, and institutional long-term care. In the past 30 years, funding for geriatrics education has been sporadic. With the exception of VA Geriatric Research, Education and Clinical Centers (GRECCs) in a few selected areas of the country, there have been no secure ongoing funding sources. Federal and foundation funds, inde-

pendently or in partnerships, have had significant impact on geriatrics education and training, although there has been little evaluation of some partnerships. The insecure and short-term nature of these funds has prevented the institutionalization of the training to most universities' education. The lack of secure and ongoing funding and the absence of a commitment by the Federal government to designate an agency with permanent responsibility and funds to address workforce needs for the provision of long-term care can precipitate a significant crisis in the delivery of long-term care, just as the scope of long-term-care services is beginning to expand.

Action Required

1) On-going Federal funding for education and training of health professionals and paraprofessionals in basic and continuing education which includes didactic and on-site clinical experiences in long-term care of older adults.
2) Use existing structures such as Geriatric Education Centers (GECs), individually or in networks, to provide interdisciplinary long-term-care training opportunities, training trainers, fellowships, and faculty development.
3) Provision of regional access to long-term care geriatrics education and training.

Responsible Agent(s)

1) Congress, Veteran's Administration (VA), Bureau of Health Professions (BHPr).
2, 3) Congress, VA, and GECs, Universities with programs in geriatrics.

Expected Outcome(s).

1) Ongoing BHPr funding for geriatrics education and training of health professionals and new funding for education of paraprofessionals within 2 years.
2) An increase in the number of GECs or networks of GECs providing long-term-care education and training within 3 years.
3) The expansion of GECs to all states; an increase in the number of universities providing education and training opportunities in long-term care within 5 years.

Faculty Development

2. Develop strategies for enhancing the attractiveness of faculty careers in geriatrics and long-term care.

3. Develop a comprehensive policy to support and encourage the *re-education* of current faculty in geriatrics and long-term care.

Rationale

One of the most critical factors in attracting students to the study of geriatrics is the scarcity of highly motivated and skilled faculty mentors. Few faculty among all health disciplines have advanced skills and knowledge in geriatrics and long-term care. The problem of too few faculty prepared in geriatrics and long-term care is particularly acute among faculty of color, and among faculty teaching and practicing in primary care. To date federally funded faculty fellowships in geriatrics have been available only in medicine and dentistry. Faculty fellowships are understood to be either 2-year fellowships or 1-year retraining. Among other health professions which provide services to older adults in home and community-based settings and institutions, funds for faculty development have not been available. Particularly critical faculty shortages exist in social work, nursing, and health services administration. Faculty in these disciplines could be attracted to engage in focused study in geriatrics if given sufficient incentives such as funded fellowships to support temporary sabbatical leaves. An approach such as this would increase the numbers of qualified faculty in geriatrics and long-term care. The success of funded fellowships in medicine and dentistry could reasonably be expected to occur as well among other academic health professionals.

Action Required

1) Emphasize long-term care in the current faculty fellowship programs in geriatrics.
2) Expand fellowship programs to include faculty in the disciplines of social work, nursing, and health services administration.
3) Provide funding priorities for programs which recruit faculty fellows of color and faculty fellows with specialties in primary care.

Responsible Agent(s)

1–3) Congress and BHPr.
1–3) Private foundations with a special interest in and commitment to faculty development and/or geriatric long-term care (Pew Foundation, AARP Andrus Foundation, Robert Wood Johnson Foundation, John A. Hartford Foundation).

Expected Outcomes

1) A minimum of ten new faculty fellowships in geriatrics and long-term care will be awarded over the next 3 years.
2) Six of these ten faculty fellowships in geriatrics and long-term care will be awarded to faculty fellows in social work, nursing, and health services administration within 3 years. 3) Within these fields, priority will be given to faculty fellows of color and faculty fellows in primary care within 3 years.

Student Recruitment

4. Increase financial support for the recruitment of health professions students into geriatrics and long-term-care programs.

5. Provide financial support for the development of special programs to mentor minority students, non-traditional age students, and students from medically underserved geographic areas to ensure successful completion of training programs.

6. Increase state and regional efforts to recruit geriatric health professions students from medically underserved areas, and to reward graduates who return to medically underserved areas to practice after graduation.

Rationale

Although students with interests in the health professions are often not as frequently drawn to the study of geriatric health care as they are to other facets of health care, it is possible that given highly knowledgeable, skilled and enthusiastic faculty mentors, enthusiasm for geriatrics and long-term care can be developed and nurtured. Funds are required to support special outreach programs to recruit non-traditional age students, students from minority groups, and from medically underserved areas. In addition funds are required to provide intensive faculty mentoring during and following graduation to insure success and continuing interest in providing health care to older adult populations. Follow-up mentoring is particularly important for graduates who return to rural and medically underserved areas in order to provide collegial support and opportunity for professional dialogue.

Student financial assistance is often the most important factor in predicting whether or not a student enrolls in and completes an educational program. Given the demographic indicators showing the exponential growth in the numbers of aged individuals requiring health care, it is increasingly imperative that sufficient numbers of health care providers be prepared to meet the needs of the aging population. Financial incentives, with reasonable payback requirements, has been shown to be an effective mechanism in the public health corps program. It can reasonably be expected to be equally effective in attracting health professional students to careers in geriatrics and long-term care. Financial assistance for health professional students who have previous work experience in geriatrics or long-term care is particularly likely to be successful, since it would support individuals who have demonstrated an interest and commitment to the field and will likely continue to contribute over time.

Action Required

1) Designate funds to support special recruitment and mentoring programs for students in geriatrics and long-term care.
2) Provide funding priorities for programs that recruit and mentor students of color, non-traditional age students and students from medically underserved areas.
3) Provide funding priorities for student stipends for students of color, non-traditional age students, students who have been employed in long-term care settings, and students from rural or medically underserved areas.
4) Provide funding priority to students who commit to return to or practice in rural or medically underserved areas.
5) Give special consideration to programs which offer one year follow-up mentoring and support for minority and non-traditional age graduates and for graduates from medically underserved areas.
6) Give special consideration to programs which promote access to academic programs for lower-level employees already working in long-term-care environments.
7) Enhance efforts to inform and educate the public about the increasing need for geriatric education for health professionals.

Responsible Agent(s)

1–6) BHPr, VA.
3–4) Public Health Service Corps; special interest groups (AGHE, AARP Andrus Foundation).
7) State and regional agencies (i.e. AHEC, AAAs).

Expected Outcomes

1) A minimum of five funded grants for programs in geriatrics and long-term care which include funds for recruitment and mentoring of students of color, non-traditional age students and students from medically underserved areas will be awarded over the next 3 years.
2) All program grants in geriatric and long-term care will include student stipends to be distributed on the basis of student need within three years. Fifty percent of student stipends will be given to students of color, students with previous employment in long-term care, non-traditional age students and students from medically underserved areas. Student stipends will carry a designated payback obligation, the exact nature of which will be determined by the funding agency.

Interdisciplinary Education

7. Health professionals should be trained in the principles of interdisciplinary team care to older adults within the long-term-care system.

Rationale

No single discipline can adequately address the multifaceted problems of disabled older adults. Interdisciplinary team care is required to meet these complex problems. Interdisciplinary teams are designed to work in a collegial manner in responding to the needs of older adults. Shared expertise should provide a high quality of appropriate care. Interdisciplinary education in cross-cutting issues facilitates the respect for and incorporation of the contributions of related disciplines and prepares the disciplines for their collaborative interactions in the workplace. Since older adults and teams are found in multiple sites, students of team training require experiences in home, community, and institutional settings. For example, within the home health setting, nurses and other health professionals rarely have geriatric or long-term care education.

Within institutional settings, there is a clear policy mandate which justifies this recommendation. The Minimum Data Set (MDS) and care planning process mandated by the Omnibus Budget Reconciliation Act of 1987 (OBRA 87) requires nursing facilities to use an interdisciplinary approach to care. Teams, including physicians, nurses, nursing aides, therapists, dieticians, and others must meet regularly to assess resident needs and to develop an integrated plan of care. On order to successfully meet these requirements, staff must be trained in how to effectively work together.

Further support for interdisciplinary training can be found in the growth of long-term care demonstrations such as the Pace Demonstrations. These programs, modeled on the On-Lok program in San Francisco, are based on this same interdisciplinary premise described above. Teams including physicians, geriatric nurse practitioners, and a range of allied health professionals cooperate in care coordination and delivery. There are currently nine funded Pace Demonstration programs, but numerous others are in planning stages. This is an increasingly popular model because it appears to be successful at keeping disabled older persons in their own homes rather than being placed in nursing facilities.

Finally, development of initiatives of the National Chronic Care Consortium (NCCC), focused on improving transitions in caring for chronically ill patients, further support the need for interdisciplinary training of health care providers throughout the full continuum of care settings.

Action Required

1) Health professionals education standards in existing professional accreditation procedures will include interdisciplinary team training.
2) Curriculum of basic and continuing education of all health professionals and paraprofessionals should include the principles and practice of interdisciplinary team care in multiple settings; educational experiences will also be interdisciplinary, with a mix of both interdisciplinary learners and teachers.

Responsible Agent(s)

Accrediting bodies.
2) Academic organizations, schools of the health professions, GECs; Foundations (e.g., Hartford, Pew).

Expected Outcome(s)

1) The number of health professions accrediting bodies which incorporate interdisciplinary team training in their standards for accreditation will increase by 50 percent in three years.
2) The number of schools providing interdisciplinary team training and the number of GECs which develop interdisciplinary

training curricula will increase by 20 percent within five years.

Staff Development

8. Educational and training opportunities should be developed and implemented for all staff working in the continuum of long-term-care services with career advancement an incentive.

Rationale

Quality of care to older adults in all long-term care settings would be improved if clinical, support, personal care, and other staff routinely enhanced their competencies. Likewise such training should be tied to career ladders and enhancements which serve as an incentive to self improvement for personnel employed in long-term care settings.

In many long-term care settings including nursing homes, adult day programs, multipurpose senior centers, home health agencies, etc., the only means for career advancement is a vertical move up and out of direct clinical care into administration. A clinically based career ladder in which professional and non-professional care providers were rewarded for increasing their clinical knowledge and skills would expand the pool of competent workers. Career ladders coupled with other opportunities for career enhancement have been reported to improve quality of care and staff retention by long-term care agencies which have piloted such programs. Unfortunately there is neither policy nor dollars allocated to institutionalize the practice.

Existing continuing education offerings are inadequate. Education for staff providing care in long-term settings (residential, rehabilitation, home care, nursing homes) needs to be available on site, at times and in time blocks which best match staffing patterns and scheduling needs.

Content must be congruent with educational levels of staff and with care needs of residents or clients. Those responsible for providing long-term care focused education need to be grounded in the principles of chronic illness, the aging process and its impact on health and illness and of the maintenance of function throughout the life span. In addition, these individuals need to have developed the ability to teach and train workers who often have minimal formal education and may not have English as their first language.

Action Required

1) Funds for training and education must be targeted to workers in all long-term-care settings.
2) Appropriate national professional organizations and educational institutions must be provided with financial incentives to develop educational materials to meet the needs of workers in the long-term care continuum of settings. Such materials have to take into consideration educational levels, language difficulties, cultural barriers, scheduling difficulties, etc.
3) Regulatory payer systems should include reimbursement adequate to subsidize training and retraining for workers within the system.
4) A national task force of professional and provider organizations should be developed to thoroughly explore and recommend cost effective ways to enhance educational and training materials and strategies for individuals working in long-term care settings.

Responsible Agent(s)

1, 3) HCFA, VA, state, and Medicaid officials.
2, 4) National organizations such as AAHSA, ASA, NAAAA coordinated by BHPr.

Expected Outcomes

1, 3) Changes within federal and state funding mechanisms of long-term care to allow financial incentives will be instituted in five of the states within 3 years.
2) Within 5 years at least two professionals associations will adopt clinical competencies within the long-term-care continuum as recommended by the national task force.
4) Materials tailored to the special needs of personnel working in the long-term-care continuum will be available through national organizations and states within 3 years.

Quality in Education and Service Delivery

9. Research should be conducted to improve the survey and inspection requirements and processes across long-term care settings.

Rationale

There is a well-developed set of regulations, most recently expanded in OBRA 87, designed to assure quality of long-term care provided in nursing facilities. However, external quality assurance of home care, adult day care, and most other long-term care services is much more limited. While not necessarily taking the same approach as that toward nursing facility regulation, greater oversight is required and there should be greater consistency in quality assurance across long-term-care settings.

In addition to external quality assurance procedures, internal quality control mechanisms have gained acceptance. To facilitate optimum internal quality assurance procedures, administrators and staff need greater knowledge about Continuous Quality Improvement (CQI), Total Quality Management (TQM), and other management approaches.

Action Required

1) Fund research on how to assure quality of care delivered in all long-term-care settings.
2) Develop quality assurance regulations which apply as much consistency as possible across long-term-care settings.
3) Incorporate CQI/Quality Improvement content into health professions curricula.

Responsible Agent(s)

1) Federal agencies; CHPR, AOA, HCFA and VA.
2) HCFA and states.
3) Health professional schools and accrediting bodies.

Expected Outcome(s)

1, 2) Findings of research on quality care will be incorporated into regulations for community-based long-term-care settings within five years.
3) TQM/Quality Improvement content in educational programs across health professions education within 5 years.

Rural Long Term Care

10. Provide funds for the development and operation of rural-based educational programs in geriatric and long-term care.

11. Require that all students in geriatric and long-term care programs have at least one clinical practice rotation in a rural setting.

12. Provide funds to support student living arrangements during clinical rotations in rural settings.

13. Provide funds for programs in geriatrics and long-term care to reimburse rural clinical health practitioners who provide supervised clinical experience for students.

14. Provide funds for the development and implementation of state-of-the-art information network systems necessary for rural-based educational programs in geriatric and long-term care.

Rationale

Rural areas have high concentrations of older adults and high rates of chronic illness and disability. Few health professionals choose to practice in rural areas. Specific strategies are required to expose students to the challenges and rewards of rural health practice. Several options are available for attracting students to practice in rural settings. One option is to establish rural-based educational programs in geriatrics and long-term care. This option would be attractive to individuals who currently reside in rural settings and plan to remain in these settings. Another option is to require that students have at least one clinical rotation in a rural setting. Both options require financial resources. Health professionals who act as preceptors to students in rural settings are an invaluable resource and should not be taken for granted. Some method for rewarding rural preceptors is needed. Examples of rewards may include a stipend or access to continuing education in their professional field.

Advances in technically sophisticated communications systems are occurring at a rapid rate. The ability to deliver high quality interactive educational programs to remote geographic settings is available. One of the barriers to attracting rural-dwelling students to educational programs in universities and community colleges is the difficulty students have in attending courses at urban academic setting. Many of these students are older, have families, and have established roots in rural communities. They are an important potential source of health care providers since many will remain in rural settings after graduation. Efforts need to be made to develop programs of study that are high quality and accessible to rural students. One, as yet underutilized, approach is the use of distance learning techniques that include interactive components. An increased utilization of this technology, including systematic evaluation and updating, would greatly increase the ability to prepare health professionals for geriatric and long-term care in rural settings.

Action Required

1) Designate funds for the development and implementation of rural-based health professional education programs in geriatrics and long-term care.
2) Provide funds for faculty to travel between academic settings and rural-based programs for the delivery of curricular content not accessible through interactive computer technologies.
3) Provide funds for reimbursement of rural clinical practitioner preceptors.
4) Give special funding consideration to programs that develop outreach or rural-based programs in geriatrics and long-term care.
5) Give special funding consideration to programs that require students in geriatrics and long-term care programs to have at least one clinical rotation in a rural setting.
6) Develop and test state-of-the-art interactive computerized curricula in geriatrics and long-term care.

Responsible Agent(s)

1–5) Congress, BHPr.

2) Congress, BHPr, PHS.
6) Congress and the National Library of Medicine (state-of-the-art interactive computer technology).
6) Private telecommunications corporations and those with expertise in the development of interactive educational programs.

Expected Outcomes

1) Minimum of five percent of federally funded educational programs in geriatrics and long-term care will be based in rural areas over the next 3 years.
2) Within three years students in geriatrics and long-term care educational programs will have at least one clinical rotation in a rural setting. Programs funded by the BHPr will include funds for student living arrangements during rural clinical rotations.
3–5) Within the next 3 years all clinical preceptors for students in rural settings will be recognized in appropriate ways for the contributions they make to geriatric and long-term-care education.
5) The number of educational programs in geriatrics and long-term care with state-of-the-art distance learning opportunities will increase by five in the next 3 years.

Consumer Education in Long-Term Care

14. Implement a major consumer education program in long-term care, with special emphasis on home and community-based services.

Rationale

For most older persons, and for most adult children of older persons, the concept of "long-term care" still evokes primarily images of nursing facility care. In order to implement the envisioned long-term-care system, well trained professional and paraprofessional personnel are needed in addition to a well-educated consumer group. Only when there is a demand from consumers for a broad range of long-term-care services will the conditions develop that allow for the establishment of such a system.

Action Required

1) Federal and private partnership funding for a consumer education program on long-term care.
2) Develop the "message" of such a consumer education program, in partnership between media, advertising personnel, and long-term care experts.
3) Disseminate a well-honed consumer education program through national electronic and print media.

Responsible Agent(s)

1) Congress, HCFA, AoA, BHPr; insurance industry; advertising industry.
2) Long-term-care experts in academia, professional organizations; advertising expertise from advertising and media industry.
3) Major electronic media networks, public broadcast systems, newspaper associations; Area Agencies on Aging.

Expected Outcome(s)

At least three federal-private partnerships will provide a national consumer education program that is available in at least one electronic and one print medium within 2 years.

REFERENCES

1. Kane, R and Kane R. Long-Term Care. New York: Springer, 1989, 4.
2. Clark, PG. A typology of interdisciplinary education in gerontology and geriatrics: Are we really doing what we say we are? Journal

of Interprofessional Care, 7(3), 1993.
3. Institute of Medicine. Allied health services: Avoiding crises. Washington, D.C.: National Academy Press, 1988.
4. U.S. DHHS (not dated). Infrastructure of Home and Community Based Services for the Functionally Impaired Elderly. State Source Book. Administration on Aging.
5. Butler, RN. How to ease the shortage of geriatricians. In Shortage of Health Care Professions Caring for the Elderly: Recommendations for Change. Report of the Select Committee on Aging House of Representatives, Dec. 1992. Washington, DC: U.S. Govt. Printing Office, 1993.
6. Health Resources and Services Administration. Bureau of Health Professions. Geriatric Initiative Branch. Geriatric Education Centers Grant Program: Trainee Data. August 1994.
7. Small, N & Walsh M. Teaching nursing homes: The nursing perspective. Owings Mills, MD: National Health Publishing, 1988.
8. Health Resources and Services Administration. Bureau of Health Professions Response. In, Shortage of Health Care Professions Caring for the Elderly: Recommendations for Change. Report of the Select Committee on Aging House of Representatives, Dec. 1992. Washington, DC: U.S. Govt. Printing Office, 1993.
9. U.S. DHHS. Seventh Report to the President and Congress on the Status of Health Personnel in the US. (DHHS Publication HRS-P-OD-90-1). Rockville, MD: HRSA, 1990.
10. U.S. DHHS. Eighth Report to Congress, 1991: Health Personnel in the US. (DHHS Pub. HRS-P-OD-92-1), 1992.
11. Infeld, D & Kress, J. The role of health administration in services for aging: An exploratory look at supply and demand. HRSA, BHPr, 1986.
12. Gerontological Nursing Curriculum: Survey Analysis and Recommendations. Kansas City, MO: American Nurses Association, 1986.
13. Besdine, R. Curricular strategies in geriatrics faculty development. In, Shortage of Health Care Professionals Caring for the Elderly: Recommendations for Change. Report of the Select Committee on Aging, House of Representatives, Dec. 1992. Washington, DC: U.S. Government Printing Office, 1993.
14. Department of Veterans Affairs. In, Shortage of Health Care Professionals Caring for the Elderly: Recommendations for Change. Report of the Select Committee on Aging, House of Representatives, Dec. 1992. Washington, DC: U.S. Government Printing Office, 1993.
15. U.S DHHS. Rural Health Professions Facts: Supply and Distribution of Health Professionals in Rural America. (CB #7590). Chapel Hill, NC: North Carolina Rural Health Research Program, UNC-Chapel Hill, 1992.
16. Towers, J. Implementation of Nurse Practitioners in Meeting the Health Care Needs of the Elderly Population. In, Shortage of Health Care Professionals Caring for the Elderly: Recommendations for Change. Report of the Select Committee on Aging, House of Representatives, Dec. 1992. Washington, DC: U.S. Government Printing Office, 1993.
17. Gerontological Society of America. The minority health care professional in aging: A rare and fragile creature. In, Shortage of Health Care Professionals Caring for the Elderly: Recommendations for Change. Report of the Select Committee on Aging, House of Representatives, Dec. 1992. Washington, DC: U.S. Government Printing Office, 1993.
18. Institute of Medicine. Improving the quality of care in nursing homes. Washington, DC: National Academy Press, 1986.
19. Hodges, J. A national certification system for paraprofessionals. Caring, 8, 2, 32–33, 1989.
20. Tellis-Nayak, V & Tellis-Nayak, M. Quality of care and the burden of two cultures: When the world of the nurse's aide enters

the world of the nursing home. The Gerontologist, 29, 3, 307–313, 1989.
21. National Chronic Care Consortium, NCCC Management, Proposed Strategic Plan, 1991.
22. Pillemer, K & Moore, D. Abuse of patients in nursing homes: Findings from a survey of staff. The Gerontologist, 29, 3, 314–320, 1989.

5

Managed Care

Ron Lankford, Lynne Anker-Unnever, Edwin J. Olsen, Janet Olszewski, Jennie Chin Hansen, and Richard Della Penna

THE STATE OF THE ART OF GERIATRIC MANAGED CARE EDUCATION AND TRAINING

Introduction

Managing care for today's elders presents providers, elders and their caregivers with complex challenges. The elderly often have multiple chronic illnesses, requiring primary, specialty, and acute care services, as well as long term care services. Within medicine, considerable care is provided not only by family practitioners and internists, but also by the specialties of cardiology, neurology, ophthalmology, orthopedics, psychiatry and urology, often without coordination. Long term care in this context refers to a comprehensive range of medical, psychological and social services developed and coordinated to meet the physical, emotional and social needs of chronically ill persons. Long term care services are designed to meet needs over a period of time and may be delivered in a person's own home, in the community, or in an institutional facility. Many elderly persons with chronic conditions wait until these conditions become acute before seeking medical attention. These exacerbated conditions are then harder to manage from both the patient's and the provider's perspectives. In order to assure coordinated, comprehensive care for these elders, the combined skills of many disciplines and professions are needed. There is also a need for professional coordination of this vast variety of services. The challenges of managing care for elders, particularly long term care, are compounded by fragmented financing. Medicare, Medicaid, Older Americans Act funds, private health insurance (including retiree benefits), and out-of-pocket payments all contribute to the fragmentation of financing the health care of older adults.

It is imperative that we meet these challenges, because the elderly are the fastest growing segment of our population and use more health care than others. Between 1990 and 1992 the number of elderly Medicaid recipients grew by 6%, but they accounted for 24% of new Medicaid spending over the same period.[1] Much of the mental health care of older adults is now falling on the shoulders of family practitioners and internists, many of whom are inadequately trained to handle these often complex patients. Psychiatric problems in older adults often take longer to stabilize and longer to respond to treatment than do those in younger persons. Two studies have shown that psychosocial interventions have improved care and reduced costs for elderly patients with hip fractures and chronic airway obstruction. Thus, there is an urgency to have the "Biopsychosocial and Interdisciplinary" models in place, to care for the burgeoning elderly population and their physical and mental health needs in a continuum of care environment.

Significant and sudden economic and technological changes within the health care system, including Medicare's rapid transition from a retrospective payment system to a prospective payment system, are being most directly experienced by the elderly. Shortened hospital lengths of stay often mean discharged patients are still in need of medical care, nursing and rehabilitative services. The delivery of these services, however, often remains fragmented. Lack of interfaces between health care and social service systems may result in a lack of appropriate care.

Managed Care Models offer an opportunity to successfully manage care for the elderly. Managed care can mean many things. The term is often used to describe any health care coverage that differs from traditional indemnity insurance. On a continuum of least integrated to most integrated, one would find managed indemnity products at one end with requirements for utilization review, mandatory second opinions and the like, along with primary care case management programs representing the least integrated models. Preferred Provider Organizations (PPOs) which create contracted provider networks, generally on a discounted fee-for-service basis, and Point of Service Products in which consumers can choose to receive services from panel providers or non-panel providers with lower co-payments being associated with use of in-panel providers would all be found in the middle of the continuum. Health Maintenance Organizations (HMOs) would be at the other end representing a more integrated form of managed care. HMOs are integrated systems of care that provide for a comprehensive array of health care services on a capitated basis.

Other managed care models include those which combine acute and long-term health care; these are the most integrated. Combined models in operation today include On Lok/PACE, Evercare and the Social HMOs, or SHMOs. An integrated approach to the delivery and financing of acute and long term care can result in the provision of appropriate care and services at the appropriate time, while focusing on the individual patient's level of functioning. For purposes of this paper, "Geriatric Managed Care" refers to health care systems that integrate the financing and delivery of primary care, specialty care, acute care and some aspects of long term care with the goal of controlling costs, improving access, and improving coordination across a continuum of services. Using this definition, HMOs with Medicare risk contracts, Social Health Maintenance Organizations (SHMOs), On Lok and the PACE replications, and programs such as Evercare are included. This paper also refers to "Managed Care Plans". This term refers to an HMO or other managed care organizations operating within one state or to the individual state licensed units of a national or multi-state corporation. Managed care programs for the elderly are designed to provide a comprehensive, integrated response to the health care and related needs of their elderly enrollees. Emphasis is on treatment in the community setting, rather than the institutional setting. The true managed care system serves to foster a continuum of care among home, community and institutional treatment settings. Managed care systems for the elderly can achieve effective and efficient use of resources. When a provider holds financial risk for the delivery of an integrated service package, the provider has total freedom to deliver all services that are needed, rather than those that are specifically reimbursable. The provider also has financial incentive to promote and maintain health and function, as well as to support and educate patients' family caregivers, increasing their comfort and competence in responding to a patients' needs. A managed care partnership such as this can facilitate access to timely and appropriate care, identifying the need for intervention before that need becomes acute. The ability to access a comprehensive range of services can enhance continuity of care and appropriateness of services provided, and foster the substitution of lower-cost community-based services for higher-cost institutional services.[2]

History of Managed Care

Most Americans have received their health care through fee-for-service arrangements. This tradition has provided patients with great freedom in selecting physicians while allowing physicians great independence in their clinical practice. This has been attractive to both providers and consumers. It has also contributed to fragmentation in health care delivery and to the rapid escalation in costs. Over the past half century, managed care has become an increasingly important alternative to the fee-for-service arrangement.

Managed care has existed for many years in different forms. Care in government facilities and the care of populations such as the military and veterans are examples of early managed care, where participants received their care within a comprehensive system. Companies that established prepaid health practices to provide care for their employees were a turn-of-the-century precursor to today's Health Maintenance Organizations (HMOs).

Several historical events were major factors in shaping today's environment. Health insurance became an important fringe benefit for workers during the early 1940's. The period after World War II witnessed the increased success of efforts to establish programs of managed care which provided comprehensive health care and combined pre-payment with group practice. This relationship between providers and members was typically exclusive. The programs were at financial risk and worked to eliminate inappropriate utilization and control costs. These plans were few in number, popular in a small number of markets, and enrolled but a small percentage of the population.

Paul M. Ellwood, Jr., MD, active in the Health Maintenance Organization (HMO) movement, urged government leaders in 1970 to foster the growth of HMOs, since they focused on health maintenance and provided comprehensive prepaid care. In 1973, Congress passed the HMO Act. The following years witnessed steady growth in the number of HMOs and the number of enrollees in them. Early managed care organizations and HMOs were typically group and staff model programs. Plans operated their own hospitals and either employed physicians or contracted in an exclusive manner with groups of physicians for medical services. The last 15 years have witnessed the rapid growth of HMOs who provide care to their members through contracted networks of hospitals and providers. This growth has led to increased competitiveness for members and for program efforts to provide quality, accessible care with measurable outcomes.

With workers receiving health coverage through their employers, retirees became a societal concern. After significant debate, the Federal government established the Medicare program in 1965. Medicare provided a rich funding source for the care of older Americans and left the fee-for-service mechanism intact. Costs for the program quickly grew and there were calls for changes in the way health care was provided and financed. Managed care programs have been eligible to participate in the Medicare program from its inception. Payment for services was retrospective and based on actual costs. HMO participation in the Medicare program was limited until the passage of the Tax Equity and Fiscal Responsibility Act (TEFRA) in 1982. TEFRA contracts provided prepayment rather than retrospective reimbursement and were, therefore, a good fit with the HMO basic product. These prepaid contracts are known as Medicare Risk Contracts.

Medicare Risk Contracts provide all the standard benefits of Medicare and often provide additional services and benefits such as prescription drugs, whose costs are usually not covered by Medicare. The managed care approach to health care can be particularly well suited to elders. They often have multiple chronic diseases and have needs that go beyond the traditional acute medical model of care. Multiple physicians and multiple illness often lead to fragmentation of their care. The flexibility provided by TEFRA has allowed managed care organizations to use innovative approaches in coordinating the care of elders.

Continuing physician education was a distinguishing feature of many of the early managed care programs and this tradition continues today. Time for continuing education was provided for the practicing physicians and post graduate training programs were established in several settings.

Managed Care and Geriatrics Today

In 1993, 48,978,000 individuals were enrolled in HMOs.[3] Of these, 2.9 million were elderly enrollees of HMOs with Medicare risk contracts. Elderly enrollees participate in 233 of the 540 HMOs in the country.[4] However, four large HMOs account for the vast majority of elderly enrollees under Medicare risk contracts. These include 1) FHP, Inc., 2) Humana, 3) Kaiser Permanente, and 4) PacifiCare. Also, the phenomenon of large numbers of the elderly being enrolled in HMOs is recent, with most of the growth in all HMOs occurring in the last 5 years.

While managed care organizations may have always distinguished themselves with continuing physician education, the history of managed care training for geriatrics, and conversely, geriatric training for managed care professionals is short and its implementation limited. This should not be assumed to represent a lack of interest. From mid 1993 through 1994, nine issues of *HMO Magazine*, a publication of the Group Health Association of America, were published. Of the nine, three included cover stories on chronic disease, care for the frail elderly, and HMO roles in medical education.[5, 6, 7] Other issues during the same time period contained shorter articles on either the subject of managed care education or geriatrics.[8, 9]

A review of the literature reveals that many HMOs participate in health professions education, and many serve elderly individuals, often with specialized programs. A survey of HMO Medical Directors whose plans had HMO risk contracts indicated that 53% had one or more geriatricians as part of their panel. These geriatricians provide primary care in 76% of the HMOs surveyed and specialty consultation in 61%. The proportion of HMOs employing an "organized" geriatrics program ranges from a high of 58% for use of a general health information questionnaire to a low of 12% for a special form for geriatric assessment.[10] Some of the HMOs with organized programs attempting to better coordinate primary, acute and long term care are: Fallon Community Health Plan, Evercare, Health Partners, Kaiser Permanente, and Group Health Cooperative of Puget Sound.[6] To further develop the state of the art in managed care for the elderly, the Robert Wood Johnson Foundation recently announced a "Chronic Care Initiatives in HMOs program", whose objective is to foster changes in service delivery, to better meet the needs of the elderly. HMOs will compete for grants to develop such innovations as new ways of organizing the delivery of primary care, rethinking the role of case management, rehabilitation services and the use of community based volunteers.

Social Health Maintenance Organizations

Social Health Maintenance Organizations, were among the first generation of efforts to integrate acute and long term care. SHMOs were demonstration programs designed to finance and provide a comprehensive package of acute and ancillary care, as well as short term nursing home and community based long term care. The demonstrations began in 1985 at four sites and were to enroll a representative sample of elderly Medicare beneficiaries in order to manage risk. These plans received capitated payments. Their success was to come from achieving an optimum integration of acute and long term care services. Several studies, including those conducted by Newcomer, Harrington, and Manton, question the success of this effort. Among the findings was the fact that the projects had few practitioners trained in geriatrics.

On Lok

On Lok Senior Health Services in San Francisco began in 1971, first opening a day health center, to serve the frail elderly of Chinatown, North Beach and Polk Gulch neighborhoods. In 1979, the program began a Medicare funded demonstration of a consolidated model of long term care in which a multi-disciplinary team formulates, coordinates, and provides all necessary medical and social services. The program has been capitated since 1983 to provide complete care to a population who is eligible for nursing home care. Services include primary care, acute care, restorative and maintenance therapies, social services, transportation, meals, personal care, hospital and nursing home care. The majority of services are provided in enrollees' homes and in the community, through the use of day health centers.

PACE

The Program of All-Inclusive Care for the Elderly (PACE) is the national replication of On Lok's model of applying managed care solutions to geriatric care, particularly long-term care. Fifteen sites have been authorized by Congress. It differs from the SHMOs in that these programs intensively manage the risk of individual clients rather than managing it on an actuarial basis across a large population. This means that PACE programs only enroll clients who have significant health care problems and are therefore, all "high risk". They enroll a small number of clients, generally less than 300, and intensively manage the full range of health and social needs. This is different from the SHMOs who enrolled large numbers of elderly who were both well and sick.

Evercare

Evercare provides a full array of medical services under a subcapitation agreement with an HMO for permanent nursing home residents. This program enrolls only institutionalized people. As a subsidiary of United Health Care Corporation, Evercare began with service to the parent organization. Evercare now has a HCFA waiver to establish programs in nine cities. Teams of geriatric physicians and geriatric nurse practitioners provide more intensive primary care services to nursing home residents than is commonly offered.[6]

Veterans Affairs

The United State Department of Veterans Affairs provides health care to an increasing number of elderly veterans through their national network of medical centers. While not traditionally viewed as a managed care program, this Department does represent an integrated health care system operating within a defined budget, serving a defined population with a closed network of providers and offering a continuum of care.

Managed Care and Geriatric Education

The Bureau of Health Professions, in its testimony to the House Select Committee on Aging, indicated that "Reports of the past five years have portrayed the health professions as unequipped to meet present and future health care needs of older Americans . . . (the) U.S. has less than one half of the number of physicians trained in geriatrics that it needs".[11] The Alliance for Aging Research reports that there are approximately 400 full time geriatrics faculty across the nation, and estimates are that these individuals spend one third of their time in clinical practice.[11] Throughout the health care system, current geriatric education efforts are insufficient to meet our needs. Consequently, it should not be surprising that such educational efforts in managed care settings are also inadequate.

HMOs and Health Professions Education

Today many managed care programs sponsor their own educational programs for physicians, nurses, and other health professionals. Managed care programs also led the way in supporting and using non-physicians, including nurse specialists and nurse practitioners, as members of the health care team fostering first multidisciplinary, then, interdisciplinary care. A Group Health Association of America 1993 survey of its member HMOs indicated that 55% of the 100 plans who responded are directly involved in graduate medical education.[7]

Harvard Community Health Plan is a longstanding participant in medical training with residencies in internal medicine and psychiatry. Kaiser Permanente, Group Health Cooperative of Puget Sound, George

Washington University Health Plan, Health Alliance Plan-Detroit and its parent, the Henry Ford Health System, are just a few of the organizations whose efforts in this area have been documented in the literature. Harvard Community Health Plan and the Harvard Medical School have gone so far as to have jointly formed a Department of Ambulatory Care and Prevention to better prepare medical students for the practice of the future.

What may be more important to a discussion of the future needs for geriatric health professionals is that health plans find that they must train new physicians who join their organizations. These physicians do not come with the skills to operate in a managed care environment. For example, physician managers within the Harvard Community Health Plan serve as preceptors for new physicians joining the organization.[7]

Metro Medical Group, which is the core multispecialty group practice of the Health Alliance Plan in Detroit, has instituted a "Managed Care College" to provide continuing education to its physicians, nurses and physician assistants. In partnership with the University of Michigan, School of Public Health and the Michigan State University Center for Ethics and Humanities in the Life Sciences, they have developed a two phased curriculum in which all practitioners participate. Phase 1 includes eight courses covering clinical epidemiology, using medical literature, using microcomputers, clinical policy making, continuous quality improvement in health care, roles and responsibilities of the primary care clinician, ethics in managed care, and communication and psychology in medical care.

The second phase focuses on clinical policy development and implementation by the students themselves. Students divide into two groups, the first addressing pediatric care and the second adult care. With significant guidance and facilitation from the faculty, the students examine clinical practice issues and how selected target conditions are managed. They then identify best practices and work to incorporate these into their daily routines.[9]

HMOs and Geriatric Education

It is assumed that medium to large HMOs serving a sizable group of elderly Medicare beneficiaries undoubtedly participate in specific geriatric education opportunities. However, no organized catalog of such efforts exists. It is clear that more attention to this area is needed. Cosponsors of the Alliance for Healthy Aging, and its participating health plan representatives support educational programs on geriatric care and disease prevention. The educational programs include some targeted to health professionals and others to consumers. Some of the managed care organizations participating in this effort include: United Health Care, PacifiCare Health Systems, and Group Health Cooperative of Puget Sound.[5] In 1989, it was reported that approximately 26 medical schools had formal arrangements with HMOs and 35 others planned or had seriously considered arrangements. In a 1992 survey by Group Health Associates, a random sample of 237 residency training programs reported that 42% had contracts with HMOs (66% Family Practice, 28% Pediatrics and 74% Internal Medicine).

Geriatric Education Centers and Managed Care Education

Several Geriatric Education Centers (GEC) supported by the Bureau of Health Professions, report that they provide assistance to HMOs and other managed care organizations in developing geriatrics expertise. Perhaps the most comprehensive effort reported has been between the Pacific Islands Geriatric Education Center and Kaiser Permanente-Hawaii. The Geriatric Education Center helped Kaiser start a geriatrics program by identifying Kaiser staff from a variety of disciplines interested in geriatrics and beginning a weekly case conference conducted by the GEC faculty. Particular patients' histories were reviewed and care plans were developed to serve as consultation reports to patients' primary care providers.

Once Kaiser undertook a Medicare risk contract, the GEC helped them identify factors that might place an elderly enrollee at risk for serious illness and expensive medical care. The GEC further helped Kaiser develop a plan to identify such individuals and provide a variety of early intervention services. The Kaiser geriatrics program is now self-sustaining and includes a geriatric consultation clinic, as well as a skilled nursing facility. The Geriatric Education Center continues to participate in continuing education programs for the Kaiser staff.

The Texas Consortium Geriatric Education Center has undertaken a managed care initiative with Houston's largest HMO, the MacGregor Medical Association. Within this initiative, the GEC sponsors bimonthly continuing education courses for physicians, nurse practitioners, and physician assistants. Minnesota's Geriatric Education Center has taken a different approach, organizing a specific two day managed care component as part of their annual five day summer conference. The two day session will focus on the goals of integrated care; differences between older people and other clients; the measurement of improved quality in an integrated model; what consumers want; and the barriers to creating such models. Minnesota will also employ a train the trainer approach to develop staff at the regional GECs as resources on geriatric managed care for their areas.

The Miami Area Geriatric Education Center and the South Texas Geriatric Education Center reported conducting continuing education activities for hospitals, nursing homes, home care programs, physician groups, mental health agencies, and rehabilitation centers that are part of organized managed care systems.

Department of Veterans Affairs Educational Programs

Since 1978, the Department of Veterans Affairs (VA) has sponsored a Geriatrics Fellowship Program conducted at VA medical centers affiliated with medical schools. In 1992, there were 35 sites for these fellowships and 315 Fellows had completed the program since its inception. The VA also sponsored Geriatric Dentistry fellowships at six sites with 45 Fellows having completed the program in the 10 years between 1982 and 1992. The Geriatric Dental program ended in 1992.

In 1992, the VA developed a Geriatric Psychiatry Fellowship Program with nine sites, and a Geriatric Neurology Fellowship program with three sites. Education is also provided for Clinical Nurse Specialists and allied health professionals, as well as fellowships in gerontological nursing. The VA established a national Interdisciplinary Team Training Program which brings together students from three or more disciplines and emphasizes skills and knowledge needed to work together as a group.[11] In addition, the VA established Geriatric Research, Education and Clinical Centers (GRECCs), which have as a major component health service research and educational programs.

HMOs and Geriatric Research

A final area to consider in this discussion is the unfilled role of HMOs in research. With 2.9 million enrollees, HMOs are becoming an important source of research on care for the elderly, and are thus contributing to geriatric education. Researchers working in or for individual plans, particularly Kaiser Permanente and Group Health Cooperative of Puget Sound, have published their research on several topics of interest in the field of geriatrics. For example, Kaiser Permanente, along with the University of California at Los Angeles (UCLA) and with funding from the Robert Wood Johnson Foundation, conducted a major multi-year study evaluating hospitalized older persons (HOPE). HMOs are also part of larger research efforts designed to add to the knowledge base of geriatrics. For example, five HMOs (Health Partners, Sierra Health Systems-Las Vegas, Kaiser Foundation Health Plan-San Diego, FHP in Los Angeles, and Group Health of Puget Sound) are part of a study funded by The Robert Wood Johnson Foundation to determine best practices in the field of geriatric rehabilitation programs.[12] The study is being conducted by the University of Colorado Center for Health Services Research and includes a total of 18 sites.

Vision

Given the graying of the American population, it is clear that HMOs and other forms of managed care discussed in this paper will become more central to the provision of health care for the elderly in the future. Whether it is a case of younger HMO enrollees aging in place, or new plans offering service to existing and future Medicare beneficiaries, the trend is evident. Managed care programs allow for innovation and will not be rigidly constrained by the fee-for-service benefit structure. Individuals generally receive all care from specified providers within a closed, comprehensive system of care. In this way, managed care will continue to demonstrate its ability to reduce the fragmentation of care that is the hallmark of the fee-for-service system. It will also continue to demonstrate its ability to eliminate unnecessary care. The accrued savings from these features may be used to enhance existing Medicare benefits by adding prescription drug coverage, hearing aid, optical and dental benefits. Achieving these goal requires the expansion of educational programs that focus on training health professionals to provide geriatric care in a managed care environment.

It is imperative, therefore, that these organizations have access to and use well qualified professionals trained in the care of the elderly population. Furthermore, managed care organizations must assume greater responsibility for educating these health professionals. The past decade has witnessed the shift from hospital based care to more ambulatory office based care. More care is being provided in the home, the community and in nursing care facilities. Managed care organizations have been leaders in this shift and will continue to innovate. Health professions training, especially medical training, has been concentrated in the hospital setting. As we continue to move toward more ambulatory care this type of training becomes increasingly inappropriate. Health professions schools must shift the locus of their training programs from the hospital to ambulatory settings. Managed care settings offer academic institutions a place for health professions education that is well integrated into the context of individual and population based health care. Quality of care and service, effective population screening, preventive measures, appropriate utilization, and the outcomes of care are important issues that will determine the success of managed care organizations. The education of health professionals must incorporate these principles into core curricula at each level of training. Therefore, managed care settings are an ideal ambulatory site for health professions education and training. The curriculum must address all key core areas and will represent a combination of both didactic and experiential training so that practitioners will be better able to address social, psychological, and medical needs of the growing number of elderly patients in managed care programs.

Managed care organizations, furthermore, often use a collaborative practice model that creates an environment in which interdisciplinary training and team building can be encouraged. This approach can improve the cost effectiveness of care through the development of prevention based strategies, utilizing the expertise of physicians, nurses and other health care professionals, as well as the capabilities of patients and the support of family caregivers. This, too, makes managed care settings the ideal location for health professions training.

One way in which this can be accomplished is for Geriatric Education Centers, medical residency and other graduate and undergraduate health professions education programs to establish ongoing relationships with Medicare risk plans. Such relationships should allow the students and residents to obtain geriatric clinical experience in a managed care context as well as having opportunities to attend general managed care topic meetings.

Because geriatrics involves addressing multiple illnesses, social systems, professional cultural dynamics, and different belief systems of patients there will need to be a prepared, competent clinical workforce that is capable of understanding the effectiveness of team practice when addressing geriatric issues. The goal of care in the future system will not be to strictly provide "good medicine" or "good nursing" etc., but rather it will focus on how the patient can manage his/her health condition in an optimal way. Since managed care systems and financing are trends that are here to stay, the effective management of complex and expensive care will require a new interdependent infrastructure to achieve system and quality of care goals. A well prepared clinical workforce to serve the elderly population will be one whose training is interdisciplinary, one which understands the importance of functioning as part of a team, and also understands a "biopsychosocial" approach to care. The collaborative practice model employed by the majority of managed care organizations creates an environment in which interdisciplinary training and team building are encouraged.

The vision for the future, is that schools and training programs for health professionals will have successfully transformed their curricula and programs to meet the challenges which the graying of America presents for the health care system. Managed care programs will partner with educational institutions and Geriatric Education Centers to effect this change. Practicing professionals and new graduates will be proficient in geriatric primary care skills and well versed in the principles of managed care. Health professionals will understand their respective roles in the continuum of care and as members of multidisciplinary and interdisciplinary teams. Most of the education and training of primary care practitioners will occur in ambulatory and community settings that are part of managed care programs.

This cooperation will provide the infrastructure to achieve system and quality of care goals.

As a result, health plans will have adequate supplies of physicians, nurses and other health professionals that have been well trained and experienced in care for geriatric patients in managed care situations. This, in turn, results in adequate access to high quality care for the growing number of elderly served through managed health care organizations.

RECOMMENDATIONS

Education of the Providers of Care to the Elderly in a Managed Care Environment

1. Training programs must substantially increase the number of primary care health professionals with expertise in geriatrics.

Rationale

Managed care and other delivery systems rely on the same health professional schools for educating their workforces. The numbers of primary care physicians, nurse practitioners, and physician assistants with geriatric expertise are not adequate to care for the number of elderly living today. The current workforce has an excess of specialists and a shortage of primary care providers. This situation will only worsen in the first half of the next millennium if nothing changes now. Managed care plans will also face an increasing workforce imbalance as their enrolled members age and more older Americans enter managed care programs. Managed care will benefit from this change and will have an appropriately trained and balanced workforce with expertise in geriatrics.

Actions Required

1) Increase the number and funding for primary care training programs that emphasize training in geriatrics;
2) Increase the ratio of primary care to specialty care physician training positions;
3) Increase the number of physicians with fellowship training in geriatrics;
4) Increase the curriculum contact hours in primary care and geriatrics in all schools and training programs for physicians, nurse practitioners, and physician assistants;
5) Provide more scholarship funding to health professionals in training who chose to specialize in primary and geriatric care.

Responsible Agents

1) All governmental agencies that govern the funding of the training of health professionals such as the Health Care Financing Administration HCFA, the Bureau of Health Professions (BHPr), the Veterans Administration (VA), and the National Institutes of Health (NIH);
2) Training programs and all governmental agencies that direct funding of the training of health professionals such as HCFA, BHPr, VA, and NIH;
3) Training programs and governmental agencies that direct funding of the training of physicians such as HCFA, BHPr, VA, and NIH;
4) The Association of American Medical Colleges (AAMC), the American Osteopathic Association (AOA), the American Council on Graduate Medical Medicine (ABFP, ABIM and ABP&N), and the appropriate accrediting bodies such as the National League for Nurses (NLN), and the Commission on Accreditation of Allied Health Education Programs (CAAHEP);
5) All governmental agencies that fund the training of health professionals such as HCFA, BHPr, VA, and NIH.

Expected Outcomes

1) Primary care training programs will produce an increased number of primary care professionals with expertise in geriatrics within 15 years so that they comprise 60% of the health professional workforce;
2) The number of specialty training positions will be reduced to 40% of all available physician training positions within 10 years;
3) 10% of all primary care physicians will have fellowship training and certificates of added qualification (CAQs) in geriatrics within 15 years;
4) All primary care physicians, nurse practitioners, social workers, and physician assistants will have a knowledge base and clinical preparation for the care of the elderly;
5) Scholarship and grants for graduate medical education will bolster the decisions by health professionals to choose career paths leading to primary care and geriatrics.

2. Schools educating health professionals should increase the geriatric curriculum contact time with special emphasis on team care.

Rationale

Geriatric care often provided by a core *multidiciplinary team* comprised of a physician, nurse practitioners or physicians assistants, and other providers who share common goals for an individual and coordinate their efforts through systematic communication. The care of some elders is best done by an *interdisciplinary team* which is especially committed to collaborative decision making in caring for an individual. These processes are particularly suited to the managed care environment. Health professional schools currently place minimal emphasis on teaching geriatrics and the team care process. This situation leaves most health professionals inadequately prepared to act as effective primary care providers for the elderly and as members on multidisciplinary and interdisciplinary teams.

Actions Required

1) Establish core geriatric curriculum content in primary care for all health professional schools and training programs with required clinical contact hours;
2) Require competencies in geriatric care including multidisciplinary and interdisciplinary team care for successful program completion.

Responsible Agents

1) Accrediting bodies such as the AAMC, NLN, CAAHEP and other professional groups responsible for establishing curriculum content in collaboration with the American Geriatrics Society (AGS) and the American Society on Aging (ASA);
2) Certifying bodies such as ANA, National Board of Medical Examiners, and other professional groups responsible for certifying graduating health professionals.

Expected Outcomes

1) 20% of undergraduate clinical curriculum content will concentrate on caring for the elderly within 5 years;
2) All graduating health professionals working in managed care will have demonstrated clinical competency in geriatrics both as individuals providers and as members of multidisciplinary and interdisciplinary teams that are often required to care for the elderly.

3. Managed care programs should establish either internal or external training programs to assure that their previously trained primary care providers have the knowledge base and clinical skills required to care for elders.

Rationale

Managed care is playing an increasing role in providing care to the elderly. Many health professionals working in the environment of managed care did not have the benefit of acquiring in their training the core information and skills required for caring for elders. These health professionals are and will be the de facto primary care providers of care to the elderly for years to come. Increasing their knowledge base and clinical skills in caring for the elderly will greatly improve geriatric care in managed care programs.

Actions Required

1) Managed care associations in collaboration with professional societies should establish programs in geriatrics with specific curriculum content and clinical contact times for primary care health professionals without previous geriatric training;
2) A mechanism should be established for measuring general competency in geriatrics for previously trained physicians, nurse practitioners, physician assistants and social workers;
3) Payers should develop a mechanism to assure that managed care programs participating in Medicare risk appropriately increase the number of physicians, nurse practitioners, physician assistants, and social workers with demonstrated competency in geriatrics.

Responsible Agents

1) Managed care associations such as Group Health Association of America (GHAA), professional groups such as AGS and ASA in collaboration with the NLN, ABFP, ABIM, ABP&N and the Commission on Accreditation of Allied Health Education Programs (CAAHEP);
2) Managed care associations such as GHAA, professional groups such as AGS and ASA in collaboration with the NLN, ABFP, ABIM, ABP&N and CAAHEP;
3) HCFA and managed care associations such as GHAA.

Expected Outcomes

1) A core curriculum and competencies in geriatrics will be established for the primary care health professionals working in the managed care;
2) 30% of primary care professionals working in managed care will demonstrate competency in geriatrics by the year 2005, 50% by 2010, and 80% by 2015;
3) Managed care programs participating in Medicare will have professional workforces that are prepared to care for their elderly members.

4. Schools for the health professions should have managed care clinicians on their faculties and provide much of their primary care geriatric training in the managed environment.

Rationale

Most health professional schools and training programs currently provide the bulk of their teaching in classroom and hospital settings. Current trends in care are moving care from the hospital to other settings including nursing care facilities, the home, and the outpatient setting. Community faculty serve as volunteers. Academic institutions cannot continue to expect all managed care clinical faculty to be volunteers if they are to play a significant role in the education and training of health professionals. Managed care programs will benefit from this arrangement especially in their efforts to recruit primary care professionals with training in geriatrics in the managed care environment.

Actions Required

1) Decrease the amount of core curriculum teaching in the hospital setting;
2) Expand the teaching campus to include nursing care facilities, hospices, and the home and office setting;
3) Make government funding of the education and training of health professionals contingent upon the inclusion of managed care sites and managed care professionals in the training of primary care and geriatric health professionals;
4) Fund clinicians in managed care for teaching activities.

Responsible Agents

1) Accrediting bodies including the AAMC, ACGME, the National League for Nurses, CAHEP, and other accrediting groups;
2) Accrediting bodies including the AAMC, ACGME, the National League for Nurses, CAHEP and other accrediting groups;
3) HCFA;
4) Managed care programs and academic institutions.

Expected Outcomes

1) The hospital will no longer be the primary site for training primary care and geriatric health professionals;
2) 50% of clinical instruction and training will take place in community managed geriatric care settings including nursing care facilities, hospices, the home, and the office setting;
3) The number of faculty from managed care programs in schools for health professionals will be proportionate to the elderly enrolled in managed care programs;
4) Managed care clinicians will have the incentives and time to teach health professionals in training.

5. Teach all health professionals the history, philosophy, and financing of managed care.

Rationale

The majority of older Americans will receive their health care in managed care programs within 10 years. Health professionals must understand the managed care environment and how fee-for-person-care differs from fee-for-service-care.

Actions Required

1) Include the history, philosophy, and financing of managed care in the training of primary and geriatric care health professionals;
2) Health professionals in managed care will act as faculty in this endeavor.

Responsible Agents

1) Accrediting bodies for the schools of health professionals;
2) Managed care programs and health professionals working in managed care.

Expected Outcomes

1) Graduating health professionals will have an understanding of the managed care environment; 2) Managed care programs will recruit newly trained health professionals who understand the principles of managed care.

6. Develop Managed Care Geriatrics Experiences for Specialty Residencies

Rationale

Introducing specialty residents to managed care and geriatric issues in Medicare Risk health plans will allow those residents, and the training programs and/or institutions that they come from, to develop a better working relationship with managed care organizations that have Medicare Risk contracts. The clinical rotations will be ambulatory with an emphasis on population-based management, diagnosis and treatment of chronic diseases, and exploring opportunities for the introduction of preventive services.

Newly graduating residents in the specialties of cardiology, neurology, ophthalmology, orthopedics, psychiatry and urology, will have an increased understanding, tolerance, and training expertise in preventive health care services, ambulatory care in their specialty, and the treatment and diagnosis of chronic disease states in a defined population. The newly graduating residents will have a better working relationship with Medicare Risk contracting health plans as it relates to the treatment of geriatric enrollees.

Actions Required

1) Funding to specialty residencies in cardiology, neurology, ophthalmology, orthopedics, psychiatry and urology, will be dependent upon one-month rotations at HMO delivery sites in the second and third years of the residency for those teaching institutions and residencies which have contractual relationships with Medicare Risk contractors;
2) One-month rotations in the second and third years of residency will be divided between opportunities for the residents to experience the management emphasis on preventive services, population-based management, and the diagnosis and treatment of chronic conditions in geriatric populations.

Responsible Agents

1) HCFA (Health Care Financing Administration), VA (Veterans Administration);
2) Training institutions, residency training programs, schools of health professions, as Medicare Risk contractor health plans.

Expected Outcomes

Measurable
1) Number of specialists practicing in staff model and IPA model Medicare Risk health plans will increase within 10 years;
2) Number of specialty residents rotating in Medicare Risk health plans will increase within 5 years.
Non-Measurable: Newly graduating residents in the above-noted specialties will have an increased understanding, tolerance, and training expertise in preventive health care services, ambulatory care in their specialty, and the treatment and diagnosis of chronic disease states in a defined population. The newly graduating residents will have a better working relationship with Medicare Risk contracting health plans as it relates to the treatment of geriatric enrollees.

7. Establish clinical training sites for health care professionals within managed care plans for the elderly, in order to develop and expand the capabilities of health care professionals in managing the care of elderly patients.

Rationale

A critical factor in determining the competencies needed in managing a cohort of geriatric patients is the nature of the population to be served. Many elders have psychosocial, cognitive, and/or functional problems; the majority have chronic health conditions. Managed care plans for the elderly must meet the complex interrelated needs of older people, needs that place them at risk of institutionalization, and must have in place health care professionals with the skills necessary to address those needs. Geriatrics requires comprehensive assessment and coordinated service delivery, emphasizing a team approach and addressing the psychosocial, as well as the medical, aspects of care. In managed care organizations, health care professionals are taught to function as a members of interdisciplinary teams, allocating resources to provide the appropriate level of care in a coordinated manner while controlling the cost of the care provided. This process can maximize continuity of care and result in better outcomes for patients with regard to maintenance of health status and functional ability, as well as reduced and more appropriate utilization of health care resources.

Actions Required

1) Establish fellowship, residencies, internships, field placements and continuing education programs within managed care plans, such as TEFRA HMOs, SHMOs and PACE sites, for training both new and existing health care professionals to work with the geriatric population;
2) Provide adequate funding to establish and expand such programs;
3) Facilitate the blending of Medicare, Medicaid and private dollars in order to provide funding streams and reimbursement mechanisms for integrated (acute and long term care) delivery systems;
4) Establish training programs for health care professionals within integrated health care systems.

Responsible Agents

1) Private, managed care plans and integrated health care systems, universities and the VA;
2) Bureau of Health Professions, VA, and other governmental agencies which fund training for health care professionals, private sector funding, including foundations;
3) Congress, public and private health care providers and insurers, HCFA, State Medicaid Agencies, foundations, American Association of Retired Persons, and other consumer advocate groups, universities;
4) Public and private health care providers and insurers, universities.

Expected Outcomes

1) Within the next 5 years, at least 30 managed care plans will have established clinical training sites for a variety of health care professionals including, but not limited to, physicians, nurses, social workers, physical/occupational/speech therapists and health care administrators;
2) All clinical training sites established in a managed care plans will be funded by designated governmental agencies and/or private sector funding;
3) Within the next 5 years, all U.S. states will have the option to develop integrated health care systems combining Medicare and Medicaid dollars; at least one such system will be operational in each state;
4) Within the next 5 years, at least 10 integrated health care systems will have established training programs for health care professionals.

Team Approach for Care of the Elderly in Managed Care

8. Geriatric interdisciplinary training should occur early and often in professional education, both within and outside of traditional institutional settings.

Rationale

Professional clinical training is focuses on specific disciplines such as medicine, nursing, rehabilitative therapies, social work, nutrition, and so forth, with a defined body of knowledge. The training is historically provided very vertically, according to accreditation standards, in order to obtain a license to practice. As a result, each discipline builds primarily upon its own knowledge and "science". While this manner of education produces a workforce prepared in a particular content arena, the clinically complex issues faced by practitioners in actual geriatric care call upon a problem solving approach that goes beyond a standard referral process to another discipline.

Goals for patient care will no longer be strictly discipline-specific. Cost management and complex chronic illnesses will require an interdisciplinary approach. A new shared language of team goals, to meet the patient's needs, which go beyond disciplines specific care, will need to be developed. Results in some managed care settings such as Kaiser and On Lok/PACE have demonstrated that effective use of resources and interdisciplinary team care can reduce unnecessary inpatient and nursing home care use, thus, producing cost savings while providing a wider range of long-term care services.

Fragmentation of services is a major problem of our health care delivery system. While a vast array of services is available, most individuals have difficulty accessing these services because of lack of coordination among services and providers. Lack of access to appropriate services can result in increased health care costs, as patients postpone receiving care until high cost emergency care is needed. Integrated models strive to provide appropriate, comprehensive and coordinated responses to patients' care needs; responses which address prevention, rehabilitation and maintenance of function, as well as episodes of acute illness.[13] Savings are generated for our entire health care system when more appropriate, often lower cost, home and community-based services are provided in lieu of higher cost institutional services. Through managing all aspects of care from preventive to long-term care, future programs may result in improved quality of life for the elderly and lower costs for the entire health care system; consumers, providers, states, and the Federal government could all win.[2]

Actions Required

1) A change in curriculum to teach communications across disciplinary fields;
2) Interdisciplinary clinical teaching, both theoretical and practical, on the management of the complex geriatric patient;
3) Development of quality and outcome measures that reflect the effective team management of a geriatric population from the well to the chronically ill and complex.

Responsible Agents

1) Accreditation bodies of the various disciplines and health providers;
2) Health profession schools, providers of education funding, accrediting bodies and managed care organizations;
3) State and voluntary quality of care professional groups and HCFA.

Expected Outcomes

1) There will be required course curricula in professional schools to understand the basis of the knowledge and values of other various disciplines and how to achieve effective communication for quality patient care;
2) Professional curriculum will include interdisciplinary learning and internships with geriatric patients, both well and complex; training in community settings will be reimbursed, along with the traditional settings;
3) Measures of quality and cost benefit will be developed to serve as benchmarks of performance of geriatric managed care.

Integration of Mental Health Care for the Elderly into Managed Care

9. Insure that Mental Health Services for the elderly are provided on an equal basis as Physical Health Care, by integrating the "Biopsychosocial" model into Managed Care Organizations.

Rationale

It has been reported that a significant proportion of elderly patients with mental illness remain unrecognized and untreated, and that when treated, the use of the medical care services decrease. The reported proportions of adults age 65 and over with mental disorders, both in institutions and in the community, is in a range of 20–30%. The elderly are more likely to use general medical practitioners rather than mental health professionals. This is due in part to the increase of concurrent physical and mental illness in later life, and the fact that many elderly will not consult a professional unless physical manifestations are present. Non-psychiatric physicians are less likely to diagnose or treat mental disorders; and when they do, they rely excessively on medication, spend little time on counseling, and have low rates of referrals to mental health professionals. Potential issues for managed health care to address include a lack of diagnostic testing for mental illness, inappropriate or inadequate treatment delivery, and lack of continuity of care. Close cooperation is needed between the medical and psychosocial disciplines, since the elderly often require treatment in both spheres. Currently, mental health services are a "carve-out" for most managed care organizations; it is thus necessary to consider including them ("carve-in") in care for the elderly, to provide appropriate assessment, treatment and continuity in the biological, psychological and social aspects of care.

Action(s) Required

1) Develop specific "Biopsychosocial" guidelines for managed care providers (i.e. Clinical Practice Guidelines);
2) Educate providers of managed care for the elderly in the techniques of the "Biopsychosocial" model of care;
3) Develop screening instruments to identify "Biopsychosocial" needs of the elderly.

Responsible Agents

1) Agency for Health Care Policy Research (AHCPR);
2) Health Resources and Services Agency (HRSA) - Geriatric Education Centers;
3) National Institute on Aging (NIA)/ Institute of Medicine (IOM) and VA.

Expected Outcomes

1) Within 2 years, AHCPR will develop Clinical Practice Guidelines for a Biopsychosocial Model of Care for the Elderly in managed care organizations, and guidelines will be distributed to all managed care organizations;
2) Education modules will be developed from the guidelines and train-the-trainer sessions will be offered to all managed care organizations;
3) A consensus group will be assembled and will develop a screening intake instrument within 2 years. The instrument will be distributed to all managed care organizations.

REFERENCES

1. Holahan, J. Center for vulnerable populations. Washington DC: Urban Institute, 1993.
2. Provider-based managed care — a health network imperative. Bloomington, MN: National Chronic Care Consortium, 1992.

3. Marion Merrell Dow Managed Care Digest, HMO Edition 1994, Marion Merrell Dow, Inc. 1994.
4. Background Paper on Managed Care Systems for People with Disabilities: Establishing a Research Agenda, Office of the Assistant Secretary for Planning and Evaluation, Office on Aging, United States Department of Health and Human Services, December 1994.
5. Wise D., Tailor Made Innovations in Treating Chronic Disease, HMO Magazine, 1993, 34(4):24–9.
6. Fama T, Fox P, Going an Extra Mile for the Frail Elderly, HMO Magazine, 1993, 34(6):22–9.
7. Haesler WK, Why We Should Care About Medical Education, HMO Magazine, 1993, 34(5):18–23.
8. Defino T, Gumshoes and Gerontologists, MO Magazine, 1994, 35(6):70–4.
9. Wisniewski JJ, Elston-Lafata J, Continuing Education in a New Age, HMO Magazine, 1994, 35(5):33–7.
10. Friedman B, Kane RL, HMO Medical Directors' Perceptions of Geriatric Practice in Medicare HMOs, J American Geriatrics Society, 1993, 41(10):1144–9.
11. Shortage of Health Professions Caring for the Elderly: Recommendations for Change, Select Committee on Aging, House of Representatives, 102nd Cong., December 1992.
12. Kramer A, Steiner J, Kowalski J, Rehabilitation for the Elderly, HMO Magazine, 1994, 35(1):15–8.
13. PACE Fact Book, San Francisco, CA: OnLok, Inc., 1994.

6

Case Management

F. Ellen Netting, James T. Pacala, Joan Quinn, Linda Redford, Joanne Schwartzberg, and Monika White

THE STATE OF THE ART OF GERIATRIC CASE MANAGEMENT EDUCATION AND TRAINING

Introduction

Over the past 20 years, the state and federal governments have deliberated about how to care for an ever increasing older population, some of whom live well beyond the age of 80 and are becoming frail. The health care system has been superb in treating disease but has been less involved in dealing with frail, chronically ill persons who survive acute episodes of illness. It is becoming clear that families are facing complex care situations, including medical problems that affect their older relatives. The challenge of bringing together a variety of health, social and financial resources to address these situations on an ongoing basis has led to the growth of case management and the use of case managers. There is a need for skills enhancement of case managers, education of other professionals and ongoing research in this important activity.

Definition

Case management is a service that coordinates and links care across health and social services organizations, systems and networks, within institutions and the community to locate and arrange necessary resources, equipment and supplies from formal and informal sources including professionals, paraprofessionals, volunteers, family and friends.

The practice of case management requires specialized skills and competencies, including an in-depth knowledge of available service delivery systems, professional expertise and community resources, to perform the following core functions:

- Completion of a comprehensive, systematic assessment of the consumer's functional and cognitive capacity and limitations, other needs, strengths, abilities, existing resources and supports;
- Development of a care plan that is based on the results of the assessment and available health, psycho-social and community resources, incorporates consumer needs and preferences and

meets payer requirements;
- Implementation and coordination of the care plan;
- Monitoring of consumer status and the plan of care to ensure that provider services continue to be appropriate, of high quality and efficient in the use of public and private resources and to revise plan as needed;
- Completion of a comprehensive reassessment; and,
- Discharge from case management when appropriate.

These functions define the process of case management as well as the responsibilities of case managers. The care coordinated by case managers includes both paid (formal) and uncompensated (informal) services provided by family members and friends. Services from paid sources include community-based and residential options. Community-based services refer to services such as physicians and dentists, home health aides, nurses, therapists, homemakers, home medical equipment and assistive technologies, social work and mental health service, laundry, home delivered meals, transportation and adult day care, and include services from community agencies, private companies and organizations and independently employed workers. Residential care options include nursing homes, congregate housing, adult foster care and assisted living facilities. Services from paid sources may be purchased or recommended by the case manager.

Basic Principles of Case Management

Case management is a consumer-centered, flexible, cost-conscious and quality-driven service. Consumer values and preferences strongly influence the timing, duration and intensity of case management and provider services and the setting in which care is delivered. In addition, consumers are encouraged to direct their own care and to involve their family and other natural support systems to the extent possible. Flexibility is required to assure that case management and provider services are only given as needed and desired by consumers. As a cost-conscious service, case management operates within a context of payer requirements and limitations, creating inherent tensions between case management's competing responsibilities to consumers and payers. Providing the highest quality services is also a key concern, requiring care oversight and quality management and improvement systems.

Principles and guidelines of case management practice have recently been formulated by a national advisory committee.[1] The principles state that case management is a consumer-centered service that respects consumers' rights, values and preferences; coordinates all and any type of assistance to meet identified consumer needs; requires clinical skills and competencies; promotes the quality of services provided; and strives to use resources efficiently. The guidelines particularly address the process components and are expected to assist case management agencies, programs and practices —whether they are private solo practitioners, insurance companies or publicly or privately funded programs—in understanding the clinical, legal and ethical parameters of long-term care case management.

History of Case Management

Since the rapid growth of categorical programs for vulnerable populations in the 1960s and 1970s, case management with its basic focus on coordination, has become an increasingly popular approach for facilitating access to information and services, linking people with needed help and managing care and resources. By the 1980s, strategies for improved methods to navigate special populations through a fragmented, duplicative and inefficient maze of services made coordination necessary and desirable. Many of these efforts were implemented with federal government funding and focused on service integration, cost-savings and improved access through a process now known as case management. The roots of case management, however, have a long history in the human services and can be traced to coordination activities from the 1800s to current legislation supporting specific populations in social welfare, health and mental health arenas in both private and public sectors.

No one profession or discipline is solely responsible for "inventing" case management. In the social services, for example, early coordination activities began when Joseph Tuckerman organized a group of churches to help needy families in 1833. Other examples can be found at the turn of the century and throughout the early 1900s in the settlement houses and a variety of charity organization societies that coordinated assistance for children and families.

Government interest in conserving public funds is exemplified by the establishment of a case management program in the mid-1800s by the Massachusetts Board of Charities and has continued through today. Historical beginnings can also be found in rehabilitation through state worker's compensation programs in the 1940s. Legislation supporting programs for the mentally ill, developmentally disabled, handicapped children and the elderly proliferated during the 1960s, 1970s and the 1980s.

Case management in the medical arena has focused on chronically ill and long-term care populations including children, disabled, substance abusers and, more recently, AIDS victims. As acute care costs have skyrocketed and reimbursement mechanisms are being increasingly capitated, methods for managing care and health status outside of the hospital are becoming part of normal practice. Case managers follow patients into the community and coordinate medically related care for high-risk, high-cost individuals.

The growth and popularity of case management is strongly related to its use with the frail elderly experiencing functional and cognitive impairments over the past two decades. Major publicly funded demonstration projects have shown that these populations can remain more independent with coordinated in-home and community-based services. A number of new models have evolved to serve elderly persons including long-term care and health insurance programs and, increasingly, private practice case managers that coordinate a wide range of informal and formal services.

The historical roots of case management tend to be as varied as today's models. While they have much in common with respect to their focus on managing care and resources for at-risk groups, each profession or discipline has developed case management for the populations it serves in its own settings. This has led to separate policies, financing, information, care and often, multiple case managers.

Similarly, training for case managers has been segmented, primarily relating to the discipline of the case manager. While some standards have been developed over the past 5 to 10 years by national physician, nursing, rehabilitation, social work and aging organizations, little education has been available for case management. The new national guidelines for case management and current efforts to develop a non-discipline specific credentialing process lay the foundation for future curriculum and educational developments. Non-discipline specific implies that case managers may come from different disciplines, but should be grounded in their own discipline as a basis on which to build their case management skills. The challenge for the future is to both integrate case management programs and services around the problems and needs of the elderly and to prepare case managers to work in an increasingly complex environment.

Case Management Demonstration Projects

There have been major demonstration projects utilizing case management over the past 25 years which have contributed significantly to the way that case management is provided today.

The National Long-Term Care Channeling Project. Several federally funded demonstrations have intended to provide alternatives to institutional placement and reduce long-term care costs for a 65-year-and-older at-risk population. Operational from 1982 to 1985, the Channeling project tested two models at 10 service-providing and free-standing organizations to determine whether problems in providing long-term care services were due mainly to lack of service coordination or inadequate funding.[2] In the broker model case managers provided the core case management functions but had limited financial authority to implement the care plan. In the financial control model case managers had purchase authorization over an extensive list of community-based health and social services based on a percentage of nursing home costs. Although the project increased the use of community services and decreased clients' unmet needs, it did not reduce hospital and nursing home use and thus did not save costs, in part because of inadequate targeting according to evaluators.

2176 Medicaid Waiver Programs. States have granted a number of Medicare/Medicaid regulation waivers in the last 20 years to encourage the use of nursing home alternatives. As a result of the Medicaid waiver under Section 2176 of the Omnibus Reconciliation Act of 1981, almost all states administer a program that provides community-based long-term care for poor, frail elderly at-risk of nursing home placement. Through California's 2176 Medicaid Waiver Program, for example, about 6,000 individuals per year, who are 65 and over, Medicaid, and nursing home eligible, are maintained at home for sixty to eighty percent of the skilled facility cost for custodial care. Nurse and social work case managers coordinate non-medical, in-home and community-based care, authorize purchase of services as appropriate and monitor delivery and client status over time. Although the program design and components such as staffing, service purchase and caseload size vary by state, all reimburse for case management services and have predetermined cost limits for care plans. These programs have greatly increased service access for the targeted population.

Community Nursing and Home Health. Case management has increasingly become part of many programs that seek to reduce hospital admissions for patients with identified medical needs. Ten thousand patients who receive community nursing care are part of a three-year Medicare demonstration begun in 1994 that pays a capitated rate for nurse case managers to coordinate a patient's care at home and in the hospital.

Nurses at the four demonstration sites arrange services and provide hands-on care. An example of these demonstrations is the "Healthy Seniors Program" in operation at Carondelet Health Systems in Mesa, Arizona. Nurse coordinators provide health education programs, health screening, individual consultations, personalized care plan, monitoring and assistance in accessing services for Medicare A & B enrollees. Program enrollees are randomly divided into study and control groups to allow comparison between the outcomes of care coordination activities. There are currently 3,000 enrollees participating in the project. Home health care agencies have also incorporated case management into their programs as treatments formerly done in hospitals become part of home care. Some focus on service coordination only, others include service delivery as well and a few are implementing programs for certain populations such as catastrophic case management following a major illness or accident.[2]

On Lok/PACE. A small number of case management demonstrations have attempted to integrate acute and long-term care. Started in 1971, On Lok (a Chinese phrase meaning "happy place") provides comprehensive medical and social services to 300 elderly residents of San Francisco's Chinatown who are state-certified as being eligible for nursing home care. Initially On Lok operated through Medicare waivers but since 1983 it has assumed full financial risk and receives capitated payments. Adult day health care and an outpatient clinic are key services, with hospital and nursing home care available from contracted facilities. Care is managed and integrated by a multidisciplinary team that also provides the care. Hospital usage and length of stays have been below state averages. It is the only on-going model that truly integrates medical, community and long-term care and has been shown to be highly cost effective for the population it serves. Because of its success in improving quality of care and reducing costs, federal legislation was passed to allow replication of the model. Since 1988 eight sites known as PACE (Program of All-Inclusive Care for the Elderly) have been operational.

Social HMOs. As another model that integrates acute and long-term care, four Social HMO demonstration sites that began in 1985 combine financing and service delivery in a managed care setting. Unlike other programs, both the functionally impaired and well elderly are served. All sites provide comprehensive case management. Case managers coordinate and authorize services, including nursing home care, and facilitate access to other Social HMO services for all enrollees who meet disability criteria. Medicare services, preventative care and chronic and long-term care benefits are included. With variable success, the sites have achieved the goal of reduced service utilization and costs within a fiscally responsible organization.[2]

Description of Case Management

Components of Case Management[1]

There is more agreement about the components of case management than any other aspect of service. The components consist of the tasks and activities performed by the case manager:

Screening. Most programs have established criteria by which they select enrollees for case management. In the medical arena, identification is typically by specific diagnostic groups such as persons with congestive heart failure, chronic obstructive pulmonary disease, diabetes, stroke or cancer. In capitated payment systems such as health maintenance organizations (HMOs), heavy use of services is often a targeting criterion. Many programs specifically target receipt of care at particular sites, most commonly at acute care hospitals. In community-based case management, the focus is on characteristics such as age, functional or cognitive limitations and living circumstance, sometimes in combination with selected diagnoses or heavy use of services. The majority of clients are identified by health care providers and community services professionals. Referrals can also come from other health care personnel, family members, caregivers and the consumers themselves. More systematic methods of locating clients, such as through the use of surveys or management information systems, are much less common.

Comprehensive Assessment. Case management requires the administration of a systematic, comprehensive, standardized assessment of the client's physical, cognitive, emotional and social functioning, as well as characteristics of the client's physical and social environment. Assessments are best conducted by face-to-face visits in the hospital, clinic or home. Assessments by phone interview or record review are quite common, though less desirable. Rarely, a more comprehensive geriatric assessment (performed by a geriatrician working with a multi-disciplinary team consisting of a nurse, social worker and other health care specialist) is conducted on elderly clients targeted into the system. From these data and other information gleaned through interview and observation, the needs, strengths, capacities and resources of the client are ascertained. This process is enhanced by sophisticated interviewing and observational skills on the part of the case manager. Professional judgment based on experience, as well as theoretical and clinical expertise, is important in analyzing and synthesizing assessment data to determine the client's need for intervention or supportive services or resources.

Care Plan. Case management requires that a care plan be developed with each client based on information from the comprehensive assessment and on the priorities, desires and preferences of the client. Each plan is developed using a standard format with written and measurable goals and objectives, service activities, a timetable for activities, sources for services, delineation of responsibilities, cost estimates, and source(s) of payment. If needed services are not available, this should be indicated. The care plan is usually reviewed with both the consumer and family members or caregivers. Occasionally it will be discussed in multidisciplinary team meetings with the consumer's other providers. A minority of programs use formal written care contracts with the clients. In some instances, the case manager arranges or authorizes services without conferring with the client or provider and no specific goals of case management are formulated or there are other reasons for managing the case. For example, a member of a senior HMO needing hospitalization could receive inpatient and post-discharge services that have been coordinated by the managed care organization's case manager according to contractual arrangements with specific providers. The nature, type, and duration of services may be defined or limited by such agreements, as well as by cost restrictions, rather than consumer choice.

Implementation. Case management requires that services indicated on the care plan be implemented in a timely and cost-effective manner, honoring client preferences regarding services, service activities and providers. Formal providers, volunteers and/or unpaid friends and family may be sources for service provision. The case manager is responsible for the arrangement and coordination of services. When consumers are enrolled in health or long-term care insurance plans, virtually all case managers will arrange and authorize covered services. Payment for non-insured services is sought through other sources. Typically, these are non-medical and are obtained through existing publicly-funded services such as Title III, Older Americans Act programs, private foundation grant projects or out-of-pocket fees from the clients themselves. Case managers must be knowledgeable about such resources to both develop the care plan and be able to access them for implementation. Frequently, case managers also educate clients and caregivers about aging issues, assist clients in making decisions about their health (including formulation of advance directives), advise regarding care or living arrangement options, help with difficult provider and family situations and provide supportive counseling.

Monitoring. Case management requires that the provision of services be monitored to ensure that services are high quality, reflect the care plan, are delivered in a timely manner which is acceptable to the client and are provided in the amounts necessary to adequately meet the identified needs. Cases are reviewed at varying intervals, depending primarily on the location and duration of the case management program. Hospital-based programs tend to review cases daily or weekly. Those located in outpatient settings typically review cases on a bimonthly or monthly basis. When case management begins in an acute care situation, case managers often follow the client across different care settings (e.g., hospital, outpatient, nursing home). Increasingly, these same case managers follow clients to their homes or coordinate with home health or community-based case managers to perform follow-up tasks. The telephone is the primary strategy to keep track of clients. Face-to-face contact in the hospital, clinic or home is less often employed, although long-term case management programs require personal contact at specified intervals. Some programs place physical or electronic "flags" on medical records to alert other personnel that the individual is being managed. Throughout the monitoring process, the care plan may be revised and refined to respond to changes in client status or, where appropriate, according to client wishes.

Reassessment. Case management requires a systematic reassessment of the client's status on a regular basis to identify necessary changes in the plan of care. Reassessments can be conducted on a schedule determined by programmatic requirements or can be triggered by changes in the client's condition. Formal reassessment takes place in only those programs that have cases remaining open at least 6 months such as the 2176 Medicaid Waiver Programs which provide alternatives to nursing home placement and may serve the same client for a number of years. Most commonly, reassessments take place every three to six months and do not involve the depth of information gathering that takes place in the initial assessment. The reassessment usually results in either development of a new care plan, continuation or modification of the existing one or discharge from case management. Discharge occurs for a variety of reasons: if the client has completed a planned course of care, is able to take charge of his or her own care, is referred to another system or service for ongoing care, no longer meets the eligibility requirements or voluntarily terminates the relationship.

Models of Case Management

While the basic components of case management are similar across programs and settings, case management models are differentiated by several characteristics that distinguish them from one another. These include: level of case manager authority over admission and responsibility for financial aspects,[3] program design variables such as purpose, target, staffing, etc., or specific program types including acute care, community-based or Medicaid Waiver programs.

An important distinguishing characteristic is the focus of case manager functions. A case manager's level of authority and responsibility vary considerably as well as in the clinical and managerial focus of case management activities. Table 6.1 shows the range of models in relation to the authority and responsibility of case managers. The clinical focus of case management may also differ based on the program setting and/or reimbursement source. Table 6.2 summarizes the characteristics of case management models.

Current State-of-the-Art of Case Management

Today, case management services for the elderly are everywhere and everyone professes to be a case manager. The practice of case management continues to grow, with considerable variation in activities and programs. In addition, several leading issues currently command much attention.

Case Management Program Organization

Goals. The goals in case management programs vary significantly and are closely related to such variables as the population served and the setting in which case management is provided. For example, a shorter length of stay will be the goal for hospitalized patients. The goal for clients living at home will be prevention of decline and maintenance of independence. In a national sample of large scale HMOs conducting case management for elderly clients, most medical directors (or their proxies) identified increasing the coordination and improving the cost-effectiveness of health care as primary goals for enrollees receiving case management.[6] Other goals cited included decreasing hospital utilization, increasing enrollees' and providers' satisfaction, improving enrollees' adherence to professional recommendations, enhancing the enrollees' functional abilities and meeting their functional needs. The achievements of case management programs most often reported were decreased hospital utilization and costs and improved enrollee medical status and satisfaction. Only a small minority of the HMOs had performed analyses to determine if their case management systems were saving money for the organization. More often, program executives reported a subjective sense of achieved savings without actual financial analyses. Virtually none felt their case management programs were costing more than they were worth.

Location. A growing number of programs concentrate on nursing home or community dwelling adults. Some health plans sponsor case management programs in both inpatient and outpatient settings, but the majority of these programs still emphasize

Table 6.1 Case Manager Authority and Responsibility Relative to Case Management Models[4]

RANGE OF AUTHORITY	MODELS
• More responsibility and authority relating to monetary expenditures and control over allocation of resources	• Case management within a prepaid, capitated system. Case manager has major responsibility for allocating resources within available monetary limits.
↕	• Case management plus control over monies for the purchase of services.
	• Case management with authority to authorize purchase of services.
• Minimal authority relating to allocation of resources or monetary expenditures.	• Case management with no direct control over the purchase of services. Use referral and advocacy to obtain services.

hospital-based case management. Although called "case management", the primary function of many of these programs is actually utilization review. However, the range and variation of settings where case managers who serve the elderly are located is extremely broad — they can be found not only in health and psycho-social organizations, but also in arenas that include legal, financial, protective services, mental health, residential, leisure and education.

Personnel. The case management role is typically performed by persons with nursing or social work backgrounds. Some programs use only nurse case managers, while others use a mix of professionals, usually nurses and social workers. It is not uncommon, however, to find individuals from other human services disciplines such as psychology, medicine and gerontology providing case management. The type of case management personnel depends largely on purpose, setting and funding. Generally, where the primary need is medical, a nurse will likely be the case manager; where the problems are interpersonal, related to family dynamics or require solutions from multiple community resources, the case manager will be a social worker.

Caseload. There are major differences in the caseloads case managers carry. Most caseloads have 20-60 clients, although a substantial minority have over 100 clients. The numbers of clients per case manager are often mandated by the payor or funder of services. Most of the publicly funded programs such as Medicaid Waiver or Area Agency on Aging programs define the caseload sizes. An important element of caseloads is the acuity or required intensity of the cases. If the target population is very frail or high risk requiring frequent visits and close monitoring by the case manager, caseloads may be smaller in numbers than those including less demanding client situations. Usually, the makeup and needs of the clients are considered in caseload sizes. In situations where there is a high turnover of consumers such as with acute care patients or short-term private-pay clients, the actual numbers in a caseload also tend to be lower.

Table 6.2 Case Management Models[5]

	INSTITUTION BASED		COMMUNITY BASED				
	Hospital	Health Maintenance Organizationon	Area Agency Aging	Health Department	Home Health Care and Visiting Nurse Association	Private Case Management	Physician Office
Services Provided	In-depth geriatric assessment; some follow through with identified problems (fewer than 3% of hospitals provide traditional case management)	Depends on plan; full spectrum of long-term care services for beneficiaries in some instances	Mostly non-service providing; information & resource linkage; limited purchase of services for low-income clients in some areas	Identification of clients at risk; referral and resource linkage	Occasional long-term client assessment service, service plan, service provision, & resource allocation; some family counseling	Assessment, service plan, resource linkage, follow-up, and monitoring; some service provision and family counseling	Assessment, screening, referral; authorization of home health, hospice, nursing home care & certificates of medical necessity for equipment & supplies; patient & family counseling
Client Eligibility	Guidelines set up according to specific program	Can be restricted to Medicare enrollees with disabilities and/or long-term care needs	Usually frail elders over 60	All ages served; focus often on services for children - some programs for elderly with health care needs	Anyone with health/personal care needs; age neutral; large percentage of elders	Majority of clients are elderly; all accepted (also focus on adult children of elders)	All ages served, generally patient/clients who are elderly
Cost	Some third-party reimbursement from Medicare/ Medicaid; much variation depending on hospital and services provided	Medicare/Medicaid reimbursement-typical monthly premium range: $36 to $135 &/or co-payment; some annual cost caps	Mostly federal tax supported; some volunteer contributions and Medicaid waiver funds; occasional fee for service	State/County tax supported; no direct out-of-pocket fees	Third-party payment for home care segment; long-term case management either folded into visit charge or extra $40 to $60 per hour	Out-of-pocket $200 to $400 per assessment; typically $50 per hour for follow-up service	Grant demonstrations; part of overhead; Medicare reimbursement for home health & hospice "care plan oversight": $58 for 30 minutes aggregated over 1 month
Referral Turnover Time	Varies-can be 1 to 2 month wait for initial appointment	Screening time varies for new enrollees, members sooner	Varies - often 2 to 3 weeks	Varies-1 week to 2 months	Usually 1 to 2 days for acutely ill clients, less than 1 week for others	Often 1 to 3 days	1–2 days; office case management meetings often held weekly or bimonthly
Professional Availability	Usually an interdisciplinary team; nurse, physician, and social worker common	Varies-usually nurse, social worker, or other social service professional	Usually nurse and social worker	Nurse (occasionally nutritionist)	Nurse/social worker provide long-term case management; interdisciplinary team approach during acute care phase	Usually nurse or social worker; long-term professional relationship; 7 days a week availability	Interdisciplinary team; physician, office nurse, home health nurse, social worker; sometimes pharmacists, therapists & DME vendors
Geographic Access	May be increased access in urban areas	Limited availability; few programs at the present time	Operational throughout country; services may vary within states	Services to elders may be geographically limited	Spotty throughout country	Increased access in large urban areas	Available through individual physician practices

Issues in Case Management

In spite of the growing acceptance and expansion of the provision of case management across many disciplines, settings and populations, many problems and challenges exist. Most case managers identify health care providers' lack of knowledge of what case management is as the biggest barrier to an effective program. Other problems include a general ignorance of the case manager's role, "turf" issues with utilization review personnel, unreasonable patient expectations and health care administrators' narrow view of long-range benefits of case management. Conversely, characteristics of effective programs include good communication among different members of the health care team, adequate support and resources, preparation of formal care plans and knowledge of the process and goals of case management among clinical and administrative personnel. There are additional issues that remain unresolved:

Provider-Based vs. Independent Service. Provider-based case management refers to case management services offered by organizations, agencies or individuals that also provide direct services including acute care, nursing home care, home chore, personal care, transportation, etc.. Those that provide only case management services are considered to be independent. There has long been concern that there is an inherent conflict of interest when the entity that provides case management also provides the direct services that are to be coordinated. The issue is whether to separate assessment and care planning from service coordination and follow-up activities. Some experts argue that the assessment and planning tasks be performed only by those not involved in the provision of any direct services. Others point to the enhanced potential to control quality and costs where the case management and the direct services reside in the same system. With the advent of health care partnerships, mergers and other affiliations, increasing numbers of these systems operate their own inpatient, outpatient, and home care services and coordinate them through case management. Many of these systems follow targeted patient populations home after hospitalization and track them in the community.

Integration of Acute and LTC/ Community-Based Care. For many years, acute and non-acute care have developed parallel and very separate delivery systems with little or no communication, coordination or collaboration between them. Patients/clients and their families have been frustrated in their efforts to navigate a fragmented, duplicative and complex maze of services. Recently, networks and service systems are being implemented that attempt to integrate information, financing and care. Case management is considered to be a primary integrative mechanism. However, there are typically multiple case managers, each representing their own discipline, specialty or department or organization. Even within an "integrated" system, there may be a primary care physician who is "managing" the patient, a hospital case manager, home health case manager, community case manager and insurance or payor case manager. This is at least partially due to turf issues and disagreements about who is, in fact, in charge.

Quality Assurance. There have been significant strides made in the arena of quality assurance and improvement in some care arenas, most strikingly in acute care settings with clinical protocols that serve as guides and monitoring points (such as patient's ability to ambulate, temperature, etc.) for physician and nursing procedures related to specific diagnoses. The quality of case management, itself, is less measurable and is difficult to assess since it is more of a process than an outcome. While in some hospital, institutional and residential settings quality assurance and improvement mechanisms do exist, it is more difficult to implement such methods with the community-based programs because they: (a) operate under many and varied auspices; (b) have diverse goals and objectives from each other; (c) target specific and different populations; and, (d) are geographically spread throughout the community.

Outcomes and Evaluation. Case management requires the regular evaluation of outcomes to determine the effectiveness of the process. Effective outcomes may include the accomplishment of goals and objectives specified in the care plan within the allotted time frames and the selection and coordination of resources in a manner that minimizes public and private costs while acceptably and appropriately meeting client needs. Efforts to quantify case management outcomes will be important if reimbursement for case management beyond acute care becomes a reality. The success of efforts to integrate acute, long-term and community-based care will depend on the ability to prove to payors that case management makes a difference.

Education and Training. Case management education and training is fragmented, sporadic and variable. For the past ten years, training in case management has been available primarily by programs that have been willing and able to disseminate their experiences. Most knowledge and skills of case managers are based on their specific professional training. At this time, a significant body of literature about case management has been developed in medical, social work and gerontology fields. The numbers and types of conferences focusing on case management speaks to a growing expertise and opportunities to learn about it. The development of national standards and the move toward certification lay the groundwork for the potential to develop formal education in case management that would enhance current disciplinary education and training.

Reimbursement. Reimbursement for case management is uneven and strictly biased toward medical or skilled care and setting; e.g., HMO, hospital and home health. Medical case management is reimbursed as part of acute or skilled care through traditional insurance streams but the range of non-medical case management has no specific financing source. With the exception of some Medicare billing for "counseling assessments" and coverage for case management in long-term care insurance plans, funding for case management not tied to medical care or skilled needs is most typically obtained through special waivers, grants or out-of-pocket fees for service. Several issues are inherent in this situation including that when services are not covered by insurance, people choose not to have them even if needed. Further, non-medical/non-reimbursed case management is not acknowledged or recognized as an important service and often not utilized by the medical arena unless offered to patients and providers without charge. Current legislation includes the potential for reimbursement of case management in non-medical arenas, but this has not yet been implemented. Until it is, it will continue to be an optional part of the care continuum.

Future Vision

The future of geriatric case management is uncertain because it is difficult to predict the future of health care. Case management must be seen in historical context, as a contemporary approach to integrating service delivery for geriatric consumers at a time when there is great confusion within and about a "nonsystem" of health care in the United States. Case managers try to connect the pieces of a fragmented system, but they also have a responsibility to advocate for changes that will assist consumers in becoming able to negotiate those systems on their own. Case managers are change agents, whether they are social workers, nurses, physicians or other health professionals. Their goal is to work toward integrated service delivery by problem solving in systems that do not currently work well. The future of case management, therefore, will evolve as these advocates identify needed changes. Ideally, case managers would not be needed in the future because an understandable system has evolved. Because it is unlikely that the health care system will be understandable in the immediate future, it is imperative that case managers work with older persons and their families while simultaneously working to identify changes that will result in a system of care more sensitive to an increasingly diverse geriatric population.

Geriatric Education

The future vision for case management requires a heavy focus on educational reform, increased quality, clarification of professional roles and relationships and continuing research into the effectiveness of case management with geriatric consumers. All health professionals must understand what case management is intended to do and what it is not intended to do. Case management is not a panacea that will fix the problems of a complex delivery system or repair the ills of a geriatric population. Case management is a process that will ease older consumers and their families through the complexity of those delivery systems and provide continuity for consumers as well as providers. This is no small task. Although in the future case managers may have different names and perform different tasks, for now there is a need to prepare quality case managers who can perform the tasks previously identified.

Education needs to be reformed in two important ways. First, curricula in colleges and universities must prepare health professionals so that case management is integrated into future practice. There are few health professionals who will graduate and enter a system that does not use case managers in some way. The vision is that all graduates of the health professions will have a working knowledge and basic understanding of case management and that case managers will be nurses and social workers as well as a plethora of other qualified health professionals. Case management is not owned by any one field. For those persons who have already graduated and are working in the health field, it is necessary that continuing education opportunities be available so that they can benefit from the most contemporary knowledge about case management.

The second facet of the vision for the future of health care education is that there be educational opportunities for those persons who want to become case managers. This curriculum will be more advanced than the case management curriculum developed for all health professions, in that actual skill building in assessment, care planning, implementation and coordination of care plans, monitoring resources, reassessment and discharge planning will be included. A curriculum for case managers will need to be interdisciplinary and focus heavily on team building.

As important as educational opportunities are, the future vision must include a balance between the honored tradition and value of professional identity and a move toward cross and multi-skilled, transdisciplinary applications. This vision calls for health professionals to become more holistic in their practice and may be discomforting to those who have emphasized their differences from others. A future in which professionals can embrace their callings with confidence, yet work together when tasks require close collaboration and even overlapping of roles, is essential to quality case management. Current educators play a significant role in this resocialization process since they influence the next generation of health professionals. Educators will have to work across arbitrary lines dug deeply in entrenched college and university systems to forge truly interdisciplinary and multi-disciplinary working relationships, teach classes in which the professions interact and design practicum, field and internship experiences in which all new health professionals are exposed to case management practice and to one another.

Certification

In order to guard the quality of case management, there must be a future in which certification of case managers becomes a reality. Not only does this provide safeguards for who enters the arena and calls themselves "case managers," but it provides protection for the vulnerable older consumer who will trust the work of these professionals. Yet, certification must not be viewed as a way to endear case management to the system, or to professionalize and legitimate a role. Certification does not replace grounding in one's own discipline. Case managers need to retain the license to be change agents so that they can work toward change in the very systems with which they interface. The future may hold a new role, something not yet envisioned, and it is important that certification does not become a way to institutionalize our contemporary definitions so that when case management needs to change it is bound by its own institutionalization. The change agent of the present can all too easily become the status quo protector of the future.

Research

Last, but extremely important, there must be continuing research on the effectiveness of case management. The newly released report on case management guidelines provides some important directions:

- How do costs and consumer outcomes vary with the intensity, duration and scope of case management activities?
- Who needs what level of case management?
- What is the effect of alternative care plans on consumer outcomes?
- How does case management practice currently vary across settings and practice applications?
- Who should do case management? What are the skills and competencies needed to perform case management?
- What staffing levels and methods of contact are most effective? What is the relative effectiveness of teams versus individual case management, phone versus in-person screening or assessments?
- What are the likely effects of anticipated

technological changes and alternative service delivery systems on case management practice?[1]

The Case Management Study Group suggests research in additional areas: How does case management influence consumer utilization and what costs may be increased/decreased by case management intervention? How do case management systems document issues so that social change in health care delivery systems are facilitated? How is case management practice culturally sensitive to diverse elderly populations?

In conclusion, the future vision of case management is multi-faceted. Educational reform will include curriculum enhancement for all health professionals as well as skill-building through advanced curricula for case managers. Educators within varied settings will upgrade their knowledge and skills. Certification will become a reality. Research will focus on multiple questions. The real challenge, however, will be to recognize the documented change efforts of case managers and to be prepared to embrace new methods as the case manager of today evolves into whatever new approach is needed to reform geriatric long-term care systems of tomorrow.

RECOMMENDATIONS

Health Professionals' Knowledge of Case Management

1. All health and social service professionals should have a working knowledge of geriatric case management principles and activities.

Rationale

Health and social services professionals who understand case management will better know when to refer, when to work with a case manager and how to accurately prepare the consumer for what to expect from a case manager. Inappropriate referrals can waste valuable time. Similarly, case managers can be extremely frustrated when consumers are referred with unrealistic or uniformed expectations about what they can do. Therefore, effective case management can be enhanced by knowledgeable professionals who intentionally refer well informed consumers. In addition, a more efficient system and use of resources should result because there will be smoothness of fit between consumer need and case management role.

Action Required

1) Training opportunities for all health professionals in geriatric case management principles and activities will be offered.
2) Professional schools, associations and centers will include basics of case management in their continuing education curricula/offerings.
3) Licensure examinations for all health and social services professionals will include questions on case management.

Responsible Agents

1–2) Geriatric education centers, educators in colleges and universities, trainers and staff development personnel in health care organizations, professional associations, health professionals, private foundations, managed care, case management and long term care providers.
3) National and state health and social services professionals and licensing boards.

Expected Outcomes

1) Within 10 years, 80% of medical, nursing and social work professional schools will have case management content.
2) Within 3 years, professional associations

and groups will double case management offerings at their annual meetings.
3) Within 10 years, national and state boards will include at least two questions about case management on licensing exams.

Introductory Case Management Curriculum Development

2. An introductory curriculum on case management should be developed and made available to health professional schools and colleges.

Rationale

Case management is an increasingly common and accepted process for facilitating the delivery of multiple types of care to consumers having complex health and long-term care needs. For this process to be most effective, each discipline should understand the basic principles and components of the case manager's role to be able to work cooperatively with case managers to meet clients needs. The availability of a standard, introductory curriculum that can be readily integrated with existing curricula will facilitate the acceptance and application of case management information in health, medical, and social service schools. It will also ensure uniformity in how case management is defined, the roles and functions attributed to case managers, the profiles of clients who can benefit from case management and the approaches to collaboration between providers and case managers.

Actions Required

1) Develop an introductory case management curriculum that can be readily integrated with existing curriculum in schools and colleges that educate health professionals.
2) Distribute the curriculum to colleges and universities that house professional schools.
3) Implement the case management curriculum. 4) Include questions regarding case management in licensure exams.

Responsible Agents

1–4) Bureau of Health Professions; faculty of professional schools, colleges and universities; curriculum developers, accrediting bodies; licensing bodies.

Expected Outcomes

1) Creation of model curricular materials that can be incorporated into existing curricula within two years.
2–3) Incorporation of the model materials at schools and colleges that train health professionals, informed with a basic knowledge and understanding of case management within five years.
4) A minimum of two questions will be on the licensing exams within 8 years.

Advanced Case Management Curriculum Development

3. A model case management curriculum should be developed for the training of graduate level case managers primarily in the fields of nursing and social work.

Rationale

The health care services and reimbursement systems in this country are highly complex and convoluted, necessitating highly trained case managers to assist consumers in negotiating appropriate avenues and levels of care. Currently there are many persons practicing as "case managers" who have neither the professional backgrounds nor specialized training in case management to be optimally effective. A model curriculum instituting a modular approach to the education of professional case managers will be flexible to meet the needs of diverse professional groups, yet will ensure better uniformity of the knowledge and practice of case management across disciplines. The availability of a model package will increase the likelihood of schools and continuing education providers developing educational programs in case management.

Action Required

1) Develop a modular case management curriculum with a teaching strategies guide.
2) Disseminate curriculum to schools responsible for advanced training of health and social service professionals.
3) Require educational preparation in case management in order to be reimbursed for case management functions.

Responsible Agents

Professional schools or organizations (primarily schools of nursing and social work), federal agencies responsible for educational initiatives in health, allied health and social services professional schools, insurance companies, accrediting bodies.

Expected Outcomes

1) Development of model advanced modular case management curriculum within 3 years.
2) Curriculum will be provided in a minimum of 25% of the advanced programs in nursing and social work within 5 years.
3) The curriculum will be available through continuing education programs in over 30 states within 8 years.
4) There will be a fourfold increase in the numbers of nurses and social workers having advanced training in case management.

Faculty/Educator Skills' Development

4. Educators in the health professions should have on-going opportunities for upgrading their knowledge and skills about the latest case management interventions.

Rationale

Faculty are the educators of the next generation of professionals and they carry a great deal of responsibility in providing up-to-date, quality knowledge. Specifically, they must understand geriatric case management in order to develop curriculum and to deliver relevant content in this area. While case management activities are conducted with populations such as AIDS victims, most health care professionals deal with older adults; the major focus of case management is in geriatrics. Given the changing nature of health care in the United States and the rapidly increasing use of case managers, it is likely that the majority of faculty who teach in professional schools have not worked with case managers or even been case managers in the current health care arena. Faculty who have been promoted to higher ranks and have gained tenure in their respective universities and colleges must constantly work to update their knowledge and skills in times of rapid change. It is extremely important to provide support for continuing faculty development, especially in the fields of nursing, social work, and medicine, since these professionals are almost invariably involved in teaching case management activities.

Action Required

1) Develop feasible opportunities for continuing faculty development in case management knowledge and skills through continuing education seminars and symposia.
2) Assure that opportunities for faculty development are compatible with university incentive systems and are valued by professional associations.

3) Encourage faculty to participate in available opportunities for developing case management knowledge and skills.

Responsible Agents

1) Educators in professional schools and professional associations, primarily encompassing fields of nursing, social work and medicine (e.g., National League for Nursing, National Association of Social Work, American Medical Association).
2) Continuing education bodies and national and state licensing boards (e.g., those responsible for nursing and social work licensure).
3) College and university administrations.

Expected Outcomes

1) Beginning 3 years from now and continuing yearly thereafter, there will be at least one continuing education seminar, symposium or workshop offered in case management at a national meeting for each of the fields of nursing, social work, and medicine.
2) In 3 years, the educational experiences outlined in #1 will fulfill continuing education credits which will count toward recertification requirements in each respective field.
3) In 6 years, 50% of nursing, social work, and medical faculty involved in teaching or clinical care of older adults will have attended at least one continuing education session in case management.

Interdisciplinary Collaboration

5. Professional schools should be encouraged to work collaboratively in designing and implementing geriatric case management curriculum.

Rationale

Colleges and universities espouse the significance of interdisciplinary collaboration, and most will find this recommendation very compatible with their mission statements. However, there are often few incentives to work across departments or colleges when it comes to implementation of an interdisciplinary mandate. For example, one university may give full credit to both colleagues in health administration and in social work who are team teaching a long-term care course. Another university may give only half credit toward the teaching load of each colleague, not fully recognizing the importance of a team effort. Universities need to examine potential barriers to collaboration and work toward their elimination. Professional schools and colleges must be supported within their broader university arenas. It is important that university administrations recognize the pivotal role played by case management in geriatric care and encourage their professional schools to work together in developing collaborative, interdisciplinary opportunities to infuse case management into the curriculum. Beyond the university walls, professional accreditation bodies can influence the content of various curricula. It is incumbent upon professional accreditation bodies to actually consult with one another so that diverse professionals are not so fragmented and separated. For example, Council of Social Work Education could work with the National League of Nursing to develop joint standards for those universities that house both professional schools.

Action Required

1) Identify and eliminate barriers to interdisciplinary collaboration within university settings.
2) Fund joint efforts between multiple schools within the same university/college to collaborate on the development and implementation of geriatric case management curriculum.

Responsible Agents

1) Faculty in health and social service professions in colleges and universities, accreditation bodies for each profession, university and college leadership.
2) University and college leadership and foundations.

Expected Outcomes

1) Within 2 years, a minimum of ten universities/colleges in the United States will have eliminated barriers to interdisciplinary collaboration as demonstrated by policy changes that provide incentives for team teaching.
2) Within 5 years, at least five universities/colleges will be funded to demonstrate innovative methods of interdisciplinary collaboration that brings faculty from two or more health and social services professions together to develop and implement geriatric case management curriculum.

Fellowships in Geriatric Case Management

6. An interdisciplinary faculty development fellowship in geriatric case management should be established.

Rationale

Fellowships would be an opportunity to engage faculty in a practice-based experience, similar to an intensive internship, to increase their knowledge. Health professionals should engage in faculty development fellowships so that there is reasonable opportunity to involve faculty from multiple disciplines. Since faculty have varying levels of expertise, fellowships would range from 3 months to 1 year depending on the fellow's training and experience.

Action Required

1) Design faculty development fellowship program in geriatric case management.
2) Obtain funding to support fellowships.
3) Recruit faculty who will participate in fellowship program.
4) Gain support from the larger university so that faculty are encouraged to participate.

Responsible Agents

1) Universities.
2) Private foundations.
3–4) Faculty in the health professions, university leadership.

Expected Outcomes

1) In three years, there will be at least two faculty development fellowship programs located at centers of excellence in case management.
2) In 3 years, at least two faculty development fellowships will have funding support.
3) In 3 years, a minimum of six faculty (three per each fellowship site) will participate in directing fellowship programs in case management.
4) In 6 years, at least twelve professionals will have completed a faculty development fellowship in case management.

Case Manager Certification

7. A certification process should be developed for geriatric case managers.

Rationale

Case managers form an interface between the providers of health care, social services and the older persons who consume their services. Case managers are trusted by vulnerable geriatric persons who need knowledgeable, sensitive and skilled attention. In order to provide consumer protection and quality assurance, it is important to establish certification for case managers. One association, the National Academy of Certified Care Managers (NACCM), is currently developing a certification process which is close to completion. Based on other experiences with new credentialing, NACCM projects that 3,000 to 4,000 case managers will take the first examination and that about seventy percent will pass it. It is important to note that certification will not replace grounding in one's discipline. Certification provides opportunities to enhance one's disciplinary expertise.

Action Required

1) Assure individual competence to perform the full range of case management tasks through a validated, standardized examination that tests the skills, knowledge and practice ethics needed to serve vulnerable consumers.
2) Develop and implement certification procedure and process including establishment of eligibility criteria and creation of an examination.
3) Implement certification process and certify geriatric case managers.

Responsible Agents

1–3) National certification bodies such as National League of Nurses (NLN), National Association of Social Workers (NASW), National Academy of Certified Care Managers (NACCM).

Expected Outcomes

1–2) Within 9 months, certification procedures and requirements will be put in place by a national association.
3) Within o1 year, there will be a minimum of 2,500 certified geriatric case managers.
3) Within 5 years, fifty per cent of community-based and twenty-five per cent of acute care professionals performing geriatric case management will be certified.

Geriatric Case Management Research

8. On-going research on geriatric case management is needed in order to adapt to future changes in health care and to evaluate practice effectiveness with older persons.

Rationale

Ongoing research is needed on various aspects of geriatric case management practice including but not limited to costs, consumer outcomes, levels of case management, various models, skills and competencies for providing case management, staffing issues, technological changes, consumer utilization and cultural sensitivity to diverse elderly clientele. The real challenge is to recognize the documented change efforts of case managers and embrace new approaches as necessary. Research should inform practice.

Action Required

1) Contact federal agencies, AoA, ASPE, OTA, HCFA to solicit funds for further research regarding geriatric case management for next funding cycle.
2) Seek funding from private foundations; e.g., Robert Wood Johnson, The Pew Trust, to encourage research that assists case management clinicians in their practice.
3) Disseminate existing case management research studies provided by the General Accounting Office, Office of Technology Assessment, the Assistant Secretary of Planning and Evaluation and the Health Care Financing Administration.

Responsible Agents

1–3) Researchers, funding sources, case

managers, case management administrators, state and federal officials.

Expected Outcomes

1) Within 1 year, at least 3 studies will be in progress to examine knowledge of case management practice effectiveness.
2) Within 2 years, at least 5 funded studies will be in progress to examine costs and service utilization.
3) Within 3 years, study results will be presented at national conferences.
4) Within 5 years, study results will be published and disseminated in practice journals.

REFERENCES

1. Guidelines for Case Management Practice Across the Long-Term Care Continuum. Connecticut Community Care, Inc., November 1994.
2. Polich, C., Parker, M., Hottinger, M. & Chase, D. Managing Health Care for the Elderly. New York, NY: John Wiley & Sons, 1993.
3. Applebaum, R. & Austin, C. Long-Term Care Case Management: Design and Evaluation. New York, NY: Springer Publishing Company, 1990.
4. Grisham, M., White, M. & Miller, L. Case management as a problem-solving strategy. Pride Institute Journal of Long-Term Home Health Care. 1983;2(4):21–28.
5. Adapted from Gerber, L. S. Case management models: geriatric nursing prototypes for growth. Journal of Gerontological Nursing. July 1994:19–20.
6. Pacala, J. T., Boult, C., Hepburn, K. W., Kane, R. L., Malone, J., Morishita, L., Reed, R. Case management of older adults in health maintenance organizations. Journal of the American Geriatric Society. 1995 (in press).

7

Interdisciplinary Education

Marie Bernard, Richard Connelly, Linda Kuder, Joanna Mellor, Linda Norman, and Ruth Ann Tsukuda

THE STATE OF THE ART OF INTERDISCIPLINARY EDUCATION AND TRAINING IN GERIATRICS

Introduction

The complexity and multiplicity of problems and concerns common to the elderly require a team and team approach to geriatric clinical practice. The development and achievement of therapeutic goals is the reason for a team's existence. But, the ability to function in a team and to assist in maintaining a highly functioning team requires interdisciplinary education. There is agreement that the complex characteristics of the older adult dictate an interdisciplinary approach to health care services. The appropriate care requires the combined knowledge and skills of several disciplines.

The demographics of an aging society and the characteristics of the older population combined with proposed changes in health care access, cost-control and quality at the system-wide and health facility level, promote a demand for education to prepare health care professionals for interdisciplinary professional geriatric practice. This chapter will focus on the state-of-the-art in interdisciplinary education in geriatrics and make recommendations for the future.

Definition of Interdisciplinary Team Work

Over the years many definitions of interdisciplinary teams and teamwork have been offered. One definition proposed by Luszki,[1] captures the essence of the team as it is commonly used in health care. She states that an interdisciplinary team is:

> *"A group of persons who are trained in the use of different tools and concepts, among whom there is an organized division of labor around a common problem with each member using his own tools, with continuous intercommunication and re-examination of postulates in terms of the limitations provided by the work of the other members and often with group responsibility for the final product."* *(p.16)*

This definition is based on several underlying assumptions: (1) the problem addressed is major and complex and no one discipline possesses all the skills and knowledge needed to address it; (2) forming a team of professionals from a variety of disciplines will enhance the ability to solve the problem; (3) individual skills and knowledge are considered relevant and equally important to problem solving; and (4) the individual persons share a common goal. Teamwork, therefore, can be broadly defined as a mechanism that formalizes joint action towards mutually defined goals.[2]

In a well developed interdisciplinary health care team, services are provided by an integrated team of health professionals who coordinate health care services across a variety of disciplines. Members of the team work well together and there is recognition that the combined contribution of the team is greater than any one discipline can provide.

Although the advantages of interdisciplinary care in geriatrics are generally acknowledged by both educators and practitioners of health care, a major stumbling block to implementation of the interdisciplinary approach is the frequent linguistic confusion. The term multidisciplinary tends to be used interchangeably with interdisciplinary, leading to a blurring of the distinction between the two modalities.

Multidisciplinary is the appropriate term when members of different disciplines, though involved in the same task and working alongside each other, function independently. The interdisciplinary approach occurs when members of different disciplines work interdependently. As expressed by Pert, a multidisciplinary team requires every member to do "his or her thing with little or no awareness of the other disciplines' work, while the interdisciplinary team process demands that the participants take into account the contributions of other team members".[3] Unless this distinction is clearly recognized, educators and practitioners may continue to believe that they are engaged in an interdisciplinary approach when, in reality, it is still at the multidisciplinary stage.

Impact of Interdisciplinary Geriatric Teams

The focus of research relevant to the impact of interdisciplinary education has been related to the clinical impact of interdisciplinary teams. Little focus has been on the team process, per se, and its clinical effectiveness in the care of the elderly. One can, however, imply the impact of teams on the care of the elderly from studies in the health care literature which have evaluated the impact of comprehensive geriatric assessment.

Comprehensive geriatric assessment, as defined by the National Institute of Health (NIH) Consensus panel is "a multidisciplinary evaluation in which the multiple problems of older persons are uncovered, described, and explained, if possible, and in which the resources and strengths of the person are catalogued, need for services assessed, and a coordinated care plan developed to focus interventions on the person's problems".[4] Implicit in this definition is the need for interdisciplinary team work. As noted by the NIH panel, comprehensive assessment necessarily involves clinicians from many health care professions, to facilitate evaluation of the patient in several domains, commonly including the physical, mental, social, economic, functional, and environmental. These professions include, at minimum, medicine, nursing, and social work. The comprehensive assessment team has, however, included psychiatry, audiology, clinical psychology, dentistry, nutrition, occupational therapy, optometry, pharmacy, physical therapy, podiatry, law, speech pathology, and the clergy. Specialty medical services have been involved in the process as necessary, including neurology, ophthalmology, orthopedics, surgery, and urology.

The impetus for comprehensive geriatric assessment for frail elderly was the pioneering work of Rubenstein,[5] at the Department of Veterans Affairs Medical Center in Sepulveda, California. One hundred twenty-three hospitalized frail elderly inpatients with a high probability of nursing home placement were randomly assigned to inpatient Comprehensive Geriatric Assessment (CGA) versus usual care. At 1 year follow-up, there were a number of outcomes which showed a statistically significant benefit of CGA. Patients who had been assigned to CGA had much lower mortality than the usual care group. The CGA patients were less likely to have initially been discharged to a nursing home or to have spent any time in a nursing home during the follow-up period. CGA patients had more improvement in functional status and morale than patients receiving usual care. Although there was not a demonstrable statistical difference, direct costs for institutional care were lower for the CGA group than the usual care group, particularly after adjustment for survival.

There have been a number of studies since the Rubenstein study which suggest benefits from CGA, and by implication, interdisciplinary team work. Williams[6] performed a randomized controlled trial of CGA in an outpatient setting, which suggested significant cost savings and clinical benefit as a result of the team process. One hundred seventeen frail elders were randomly assigned to CGA versus usual care by a community internist. Baseline assessment revealed no significant differences between the CGA patients and the usual care patients. During a 1 year follow-up period, however, CGA patients had 23 hospitalizations and 67- hospital days versus 23 admissions and 1113 hospital days for the usual care patients. Annual hospital costs averaged $4,297 for CGA subjects versus $7,018 for controls. Although none of theses differences were statistically significant, they suggest that in a larger cohort, significant cost savings from CGA (and by implication, interdisciplinary teams), would be evident.

Several have argued that the benefit of CGA is merely the focus upon the several domains of function of frail elders—physical, psychological, and social. This would imply that the interdisciplinary team has no impact upon the outcome of CGA. Rubenstein[7] demonstrated, however, that applying the tools of CGA without the team is not necessarily effective. Seventy-six UCLA clinical volunteer faculty in community office practices were randomly assigned to experimental and control groups with the experimental group of physicians receiving education in the use of CGA tools. A total of 510 patients with functional disabilities, who visited the physicians in this study at least four times a year, were subsequently evaluated over a 1 year period. Forty-three percent of experimental physicians reported the use of tools from CGA. There were no discernible differences, however, in the outcomes of patients cared for by the experimental physicians versus control physicians. In subsequent discussion, it was noted that the educational intervention provided the experimental physicians was aimed at helping physicians themselves to change patient function. The authors postulate that study results may have shown a beneficial impact of the education had the education focused on referral to other members of an interdisciplinary team, such that interdisciplinary team interaction might occur. In spite of the experimental physicians in this study being favorably inclined towards the tools of CGA, one discipline, medicine, in this case did not have a significant impact on patient outcomes. A more recent follow-up study by the same group yielded similar findings.[8]

The challenge of demonstrating the efficacy of CGA, and interdisciplinary team interactions, is the fact that teams have diverse compositions, ranging from the basic team defined above in the NIH consensus statement, to very elaborate teams of eight, ten, or more members representing different professions. In a recent supplement to the Journal of the American Geriatrics Society, a meta-analysis was performed of the impact of CGA by Rubenstein.[9] All published controlled trials involving CGA coupled with some therapy (geriatric evaluation and management, GEM) were pooled to evaluate a single outcome; mortality. Trials were grouped in four areas: inpatient consultation services, inpatient GEM units, home assessment services, and outpatient GEM programs. Analysis of 6-month mortality demonstrated no significant survival effect was found for outpatient GEM programs. There was, however, a 39% reduction of mortality for inpatient consultation services; a 37% reduction of mortality with inpatient GEM units; and a 29% reduction of mortality for home assessments. Given the 1989 Rubenstein report, it can be assumed that team interactions play a significant role in patient outcomes.

Interdisciplinary teams do have a positive impact on individual members. Team meetings provide a legitimate formal means for health care professionals to come together to share insights and frustrations and to gather strength from each other in the form of professional support and recognition. Studies in the early 1980's[10, 11, 12] found that health care professionals who were members of an interdisciplinary team possessed higher levels of morale and job satisfaction than those who were non-team participants. Recent studies of social workers as members of interdisciplinary teams have resulted in similar findings. Poulin,[13] in surveying over eight hundred social workers, noted that team members controlled their job roles significantly more than those not on teams, contributing to the higher morale. Mellor[14] observed that team meetings provide a respite for participants from the patient/client issues that wait beyond the doors of the meeting rooms. Team meetings also offer opportunities for informal contacts and feedback between the disciplines concerning patient care which is unrelated to the specific cases scheduled for discussion. The meetings allow ease of access to each other and reduce the time needed for health care professionals to connect with each other concerning patient care.

More research is needed to evaluate the impact of interdisciplinary teams. Present data suggests, however, a beneficial clinical impact for both patient and health care professionals involved in interdisciplinary teams. It is highly probable that interdisciplinary team care for the elderly will prove more cost-effective than traditional medical approaches.

History

Interest in interdisciplinary health care teams is not new. Early efforts began in the late 1940's and early 1950's with the work of Martin Cherasky and George Silver, physicians who advocated a team approach to delivering primary care services. Members of the team were often identified as the physician, nurse, and social worker who worked together caring for families, emphasizing the provision of health services and prevention.

During the 1960's, interest in interdisciplinary education grew as the Student American Medical Association challenged the traditional methods of medical education. Under its leadership interdisciplinary education experiences were developed for students from medicine and other health professions.

In this same time period the federal government played a key role in the development of interdisciplinary teams when it advocated the use of health teams in its newly created Neighborhood Health Center program, under the auspices of the Office of Economic Opportunity. Team activities at one such center, the Martin Luther King Community Health Center was documented in one of the best known early books on health care teams, *Making Health Care Teams Work.*[15] Another book, *The Team Approach to Primary Care*[16] provided a summary of many of the early team efforts. Interest in health care teams continued at the federal level with the Health Manpower Educational Initiatives Awards (HMEIA) which furnished funds to a number of medical schools and universities to develop model interdisciplinary health team training programs during the mid 1970's.

The Bureau of Health Professions began funding interdisciplinary education in the mid 1970's. The Bureau has continued an interest in this aspect of education and remains a major contributor in the development of interdisciplinary education. Currently, the Bureau provides funding for the development of rural interdisciplinary training and promotes interdisciplinary geriatric education through Geriatric Education Centers.

Both the Robert Wood Johnson and W.K. Kellogg Foundations provided resources for innovative educational programs. These private foundations were interested in the development of interdisciplinary experiences for students in the health professions which emphasized interdisciplinary collaboration and the development of health care teams.

In 1975 the Department of Veteran Affairs funded several Health Manpower grants related to interdisciplinary education. One of these, at the University of Wisconsin-Madison and the VA Medical Center focused on developing interdisciplinary teams to deliver geriatric care. Later, in 1979, the VA continued its commitment to geriatric education by developing the Interdisciplinary Team Training in Geriatrics Program (ITTG) as one of the cornerstone programs in its commitment to educating staff and students about the needs of aging veterans and the field of geriatrics. The unique aspect of the ITTG was that it focused on education in geriatrics and teamwork. Twelve model programs now exist and continue to provide training for hundreds of VA personnel.

By the 1980's, the availability of grants for interdisciplinary programs markedly declined and the number of programs offering interdisciplinary education for health professional students significantly decreased. As financial resources became scarcer, universities and medical schools failed to continue to support these programs and few continued to exist. The VA and the Bureau, however, continue their strong support of interdisciplinary geriatric education.

Present Status

Constraints

In spite of the overwhelming need for interdisciplinary functioning in the assessment and care of the older patient and, consequently, for an interdisciplinary approach to geriatric education, there are several barriers and constraints. Experienced in both clinical and educational settings, some of these constraints are specific and others are more barriers of perception than reality, but all may hinder the interdisciplinary approach.

1. Differences Between the Disciplines.

Innate differences between the disciplines can interfere with interdisciplinary collaboration. These differences are identified as:

A. *Culture and Philosophy of Each Discipline.* Every discipline has its own culture which includes a philosophy towards geriatric patient care. The differing emphases can create misunderstandings and lack of sympathy by members of one discipline towards the members of another discipline. The culture also results in a specific language or jargon which each discipline utilizes as an inside means of shorthand communication. When members of more than one discipline come together on an issue, the differences in professional languages cause frustration at best and genuine misunderstandings at worse. The same words and phrases can mean totally different things to different disciplines and until the members of the disciplines become familiar with these different nuances of meaning, difficulties will arise in both clinical and educational settings.

B. *Varying Qualifications.* Required qualifications for health care disciplines vary and can range from doctoral or fellow status to a bachelor's degree or paraprofessional training. The differential status that is assigned by society because of educational attainment can influence interdisciplinary sharing and team collegiality, resulting in power and leadership between the disciplines being dependent on discipline rather than specific knowledge, expertise or familiarity with the specific patient case under review.

C. *Scheduling and Time Constraints.* Health care professionals follow busy and full schedules within their own discipline's parameters and finding time to engage in interdisciplinary contacts may be problematic, especially when the various disciplines tend to follow different scheduling patterns. Similarly in the educational setting, different disciplines may follow disparate academic calendars and educational schedules, making interdisciplinary teaching difficult to arrange so that it meshes appropriately with each discipline's educational format.

2. Turf Issues.

Each discipline possesses a unique body of knowledge and area of expertise. Interdisciplinary geriatric care threatens the status quo, requiring, as it does, a sharing of information and potential relinquishing of individual authority to others, on behalf of the older patient. For those involved in an interdisciplinary team relationship there is a constant "push-pull" tension. On one hand, the individual wants members of other disciplines to understand his/her special expertise but on the other hand, too much familiarity with the discipline specific knowledge base, means an encroachment on a discipline's turf and may be resented. Each discipline is rightfully proud of its unique knowledge and skill base but therein lies the danger of assuming that those from other disciplines are not equally competent in their own discipline. Faulkner[17] refers to this as "disciplinary ethnocentrism." Turf issues within academia are exacerbated by the uncertainty as to which professional school "owns" the students in an interdisciplinary class. If students are taught interdisciplinary knowledge and skills within their own discipline this difficulty may not arise but once students from several disciplines are brought together to be taught and to teach each other, turf battles may escalate to an argument concerning which department/school receives tuition fees and which department/school awards credit. Professional education is currently discipline specific and any alterations from this causes difficulties and requires system changes.

3. Administrative Resistance.
In the practice setting, interdisciplinary care, in particular, interdisciplinary team activity requires administrative sanction and support. Without such support, the interdisciplinary team will face difficulties in gaining the necessary collaboration from the systems within the acute care or long term care facility. This collaboration is needed for the care plan to be carried out.

Similarly, administrative support is necessary for interdisciplinary education to occur within the academic setting. Without the support of a school's administrators—President, Deans, and Department Chairs—faculty will not be afforded the opportunity and time to work collaboratively with faculty from other disciplines and any existing problems between schools and departments will act as barriers to interdisciplinary activities. Hence administrative resistance, or even indifference, poses a real constraint to the growth of the interdisciplinary approach.

Constraints Specific to the Practice Setting

1. Locations and Schedules.
In the practice setting, health care professionals may divide their time between various locations; the acute-care setting and the private office; the outpatient clinic and the long-term-care facility, etcetera. The logistics of bringing the disciplines together for team meetings or even to engage in telephone contacts can be daunting.

2. Patient Care Priorities.
Clinical demands may clash with interdisciplinary team demands and under these circumstances, priority is given to patient care. Even if structured, established times are set aside for interdisciplinary team meetings, team members may be called away from deliberations and interdisciplinary collaboration if patient needs warrant. This is particularly evident in the acute-care setting where there time is constrained for diagnosis and treatment decisions because of the nature of patient population problems and system demands.

3. Reimbursement Issues.
Third party reimbursement for geriatric health care is related to the work activities of specific disciplines. In most instances, time taken for interdisciplinary care, team meetings, etc. are not considered reimbursable.

Constraints Specific to the Educational Setting

1. Lack of Faculty and Clinical Role Models.
A very real barrier to interdisciplinary education in geriatrics is the paucity of educators qualified to teach this knowledge base. There is also a lack of clinicians who practice interdisciplinary geriatric care and who can be role models for students.

2. Lack of Clinical Education Sites.
To be effective, interdisciplinary education must include on-site clinical education as well as classroom teaching. Although clinical sites may involve representatives of different disciplines working together there is

a shortage of clinical sites where interdisciplinary team work is practiced. Discipline-specific professional schools do not, at present, look for this characteristic in establishing partnerships for clinical education of their students.

3. Lack of Curricula.
There is a scarcity of curricula in interdisciplinary geriatric care. There are some beginning curricular efforts and a growing body of literature on suggested content to be incorporated into any curriculum, but overall few interdisciplinary courses or curriculum content areas have been developed and evaluated.

4. Ownership and Recognition.
One of the reasons for the paucity of curriculum development is that it is unclear which discipline, if any, "owns" the curriculum. By its very nature, the content cuts across disciplines and no one discipline may legitimately lay claim to ownership. This results in a lack of leadership by any one discipline in taking responsibility for curriculum development or even bringing together an academic interdisciplinary team to construct curriculum guidelines and content. Related to this is the fact that specific disciplines in the academic setting tend to not offer credit or recognition for involvement of their faculty in interdisciplinary educational activities. Interdisciplinary work by faculty is rarely considered applicable for attainment of tenure or given equal value to similar work and contributions within the individual's own discipline.

In spite of these constraints to the growth of interdisciplinary care and education, there is a firm belief by health care professionals that geriatric care requires an interdisciplinary approach. Literature in the past has focused on constraints solely as an attempt to understand how interdisciplinary care and education can be most effectively established. Currently there are a number of trends and developments in health care in the U.S. that are counteracting the constraints and offer a favorable climate for the future of interdisciplinary geriatric care.

Opportunities

Several trends and emerging interests not only support the need for interdisciplinary geriatric care but offer a milieu which is especially favorable to its advancement.

1. Health Maintenance Organizations (HMOs) and Managed Care.
The growth in health networks and health maintenance organizations is a response in part, to the high cost of health care and the need to increase efficiency and prevent duplication. Health networks are extremely conducive to interdisciplinary care. Health insurance plans, linking an individual to a defined network of health services and practitioners, aim to control costs, manage appropriate use of care, and enable a health care consumer to move within the system between health care professionals and settings as care needs warrant. To be effective in this HMO role, easy communication between the various components of the health maintenance organization, the care providers from all disciplines, and the individual patient and the family is required. The flow of information and the communication modalities that are currently arising assist in bringing members of different disciplines together, create innovative channels for dialogue and emphasize the value of professional interaction as part of a larger team effort.

These approaches presuppose a group of

professionals trained at a variety of levels and well-acquainted with the roles and responsibilities of other professionals in the system. The increased emphasis on primary care and community health needs as advocated in the 1991 Pew Foundation report,[18] also expands the need for coordinated care delivery and promotes the development of new roles and responsibilities for mid-level health professionals. This increasing emphasis on community needs is also reflected in proposals at the federal level expanding the role of states in establishing requirements at the state level.

2. Emphasis on Health Promotion.
The Healthy People 2000 initiative is an outward manifestation of the current emphasis on preventive care for all ages. Studies reveal that preventive care can, in many cases, avoid the high cost of potential future care and thus administrators, the insurance industry and policy planners are fostering a redirection towards health maintenance and avoidance of lifestyles that result in poor health. This comparatively new emphasis on preventive care, at all ages and at every level of health, is predicated on activities to facilitate early detection of potential health problems and the encouragement of individual responsibility for personal well-being through nutrition, exercise, stress reduction and avoidance of drugs, alcohol and tobacco. This new direction necessarily involves a range of health care professionals. Routine diagnostic tests may be administered by technicians and interpreted by specialists, involving additional health care providers. Interaction and communication between the various disciplines on behalf of each individual is crucial to management of health promotion, and the interdisciplinary team approach is the logical means of assuring this.

3. Case Management.
Closely allied with the trends toward health networks, managed care and preventive care is the interest and growth in case management. This is especially true for the geriatric population. The tendency for the older person to experience chronic health conditions and the interplay of two or more conditions with the normal aging process has already been identified as resulting in a need for careful integration of health care decisions and management. This, in turn, has led to the rise of the phenomena of case managers—health care professionals who act as the coordinator, advocate, advisor, for the older patient and their family in accessing and utilizing appropriate health and social services. Case managers act as the coordinator of services and are responsible for communication between the various service providers on behalf of the individual patient. Interdisciplinary geriatric care is at the heart of the work they undertake.

4. Continuous Quality Improvement (CQI).
Developing and providing comprehensive services to meet the needs of geriatric populations and improve their quality of life is currently a goal for healthcare organizations. Historically, efforts to maintain quality of healthcare programs and services had taken the form of determining utilization of the service and whether it met a minimal standard of quality. Measures to continually improve the quality of care or services, however, were episodic parts of the program whereby a new quality standard was set. Currently, quality assurance programs within healthcare systems have evolved into quality improvement programs in order to meet the changing needs of the patients and to provide a mechanism for continuous improvement related to patient outcomes.

The use of continual quality improvement methods/measures have recently been mandated for healthcare organizations by the Joint Commission for Accreditation of Healthcare Organizations.[19] The emphasis on quality improvement in health care evolved from the revolutionary changes produced in business and industry when quality improvement methodology was introduced. The continuous improvement approach augments the healthcare providers' ability by combining knowledge and skills for improvement with their discipline specific knowledge.

The continual improvement process focuses on analyzing the system of service delivery, breaking it down into the component parts (processes) and then identifying the points at which interventions can make a substantial difference.[20] Emphasis is placed on improving the processes and setting new levels for standard performance or outcomes, then monitoring the processes for achievement of the standard or outcomes which creates a mechanism for continual improvement. Therefore, continual improvement focuses on constantly improving a system rather than only monitoring the system for compliance with a quality standard which was characteristic of traditional quality assurance programs.

In order to implement continual quality improvement in healthcare, interdisciplinary teams must be formed to analyze the completed processes involved in patient care systems. In order to understand the systems and processes associated with health care delivery, information should be derived from all of the people involved in patient care, thereby necessitating an interdisciplinary team composed of both the direct care providers and those influenced by the clinical decisions.

Measurement of outcomes in healthcare using continual improvement methodology focuses not only on the immediate clinical outcome, but also on the patient's overall health status, associated costs, and satisfaction of those affected by the healthcare delivery system. The use of CQI methods within geriatric services holds promise for improving patient outcomes while considering the cost of health care delivery. Because continual improvement methodology is becoming an integral process of health care organizations, it is imperative that health professional students receive education in its use as a part of their academic curricula in geriatric care.

5. U.S. Department of Veterans Affairs. In 1979, the Interdisciplinary Team Training in Geriatrics Program (ITTG) was established to provide leadership in interdisciplinary education/training using a team approach to service delivery throughout the VA system. Twelve model programs continue to serve as a resource for clinically based educational experiences for VA employees and affiliated students from a variety of disciplines. When initiated, the program focused exclusively on geriatric programs, but recently its name was changed to the Interdisciplinary Team Training Program (ITTP) to reflect a broader population served by the program. The emphasis on geriatrics is still maintained, and over 60 clinical teams have been formed and 5,000 VA personnel trained in teamwork.[2] The VA is recognized for its national leadership in the development of interdisciplinary teams and the contributions VA staff make towards research and education in this area.

6. Bureau of Health Professions, HRSA. The Bureau of Health Professions within the Health Resource and Services Administration (HRSA) actively promotes the philosophy of interdisciplinary geriatric care

and mandates interdisciplinary approaches for many of the training programs the Bureau funds.

In 1983, the Bureau funded four Geriatric Education Centers (GECs) and building on the success of these centers, has since funded a total of 50 different centers. Currently, twenty GECs are receiving funding. The GECs are mandated to provide geriatric education to health care professionals, one condition of funding being that a minimum of four different disciplines be targeted for education. As a result, the GECs have become centers which promote interdisciplinary geriatric education, bringing members of many disciplines together to learn and share information, and producing articles and curriculum on interdisciplinary geriatric care and team modalities.

The Interdisciplinary Training for Health Care for Rural Areas grant program, administered by HRSA, was authorized in 1988. The first projects were funded in 1990 as a mechanism for encouraging health care professionals to practice in rural communities. Of the 30 projects funded since its inception, twenty-two identify the undeserved, rural, geriatric population as a specific target group. A variety of interdisciplinary education models, involving a broad range of health professionals and provider organizations, have been developed through this program.

The Geriatric Medicine and Dentistry Fellowship programs, and the Geriatric Nurse Practitioner and Gero-Psychiatric Nurse programs also are administered by HRSA. All these programs include an emphasis on interdisciplinary training and patient care.

7. Federal and State Regulations.
The Omnibus Budget Reconciliation Act of '87 (OBRA) introduced a number of regulations for nursing home care which are based on quality of life issues and designed to ensure a minimum standard of quality care throughout the U.S. Among the regulations, which duplicate regulations adopted by several states to varying degrees, are guidelines governing the assessment and care plans for nursing home residents. Health care professionals from different disciplines are required to develop treatment goals and to report progress on a regular basis. This has encouraged nursing home facilities to develop interdisciplinary teams to fulfill these requirements in a timely fashion.

8. Joint Commission for Accreditation of Healthcare Organizations (JCAHO).
The 1994 standards of the JCAHO emphasizes an interdisciplinary approach to providing patient care. The standards require that teams representing the disciplines involved in the care of the client demonstrate their improvement of performance and level of quality care. In order for hospitals and other health care organizations to be compliant with the standards, multi or interdisciplinary teams must be operational. Health care professionals being educated to provide care under the new JCAHO standards must possess the knowledge and skills to be able to participate in interdisciplinary teams.

Current health care trends and the work already begun on behalf of interdisciplinary geriatric education provide a firm foundation for increased initiatives in this arena, while the recommendations at the end of this chapter offer means of overcoming or removing the recognized barriers.

The opportunities for interdisciplinary practice cannot be met effectively without appropriate education of health professions students and growth and development through interdisciplinary continuing education opportunities. A number of trends occurring in health professions education, such as problem-based learning, electronic-based information technology and population-based education based on the goals of Healthy People 2000 are also reinforcing a move toward interdisciplinary education in the health professions.

Definition of Interdisciplinary Education

The term interdisciplinary education is used to describe a process which encourages the integration of different perspectives on a defined subject. Usually a firm foundation for interdisciplinary education is introduced by a single faculty member teaching students from a single profession or discipline. Although the process of interdisciplinary education may take many forms, three models are most often used: a teacher from one discipline teaching students from a variety of disciplines; a team of teachers from multiple disciplines working with students from a single discipline; or ideally a team of teachers from different disciplines instructing a group of students from more than one discipline. In each of these cases, the goal remains the same: to expose students to a shared knowledge base so that they gain a basic understanding of the core concepts, principles, and contributions of a variety of disciplines.

Academic Requirements

Curriculum requirements for medicine, nursing and social work as specified by the accrediting bodies do not specifically mandate that separate courses in the areas of geriatrics or interdisciplinary education be included. The terminal competencies for the graduates of all three disciplines require, however, that they posses a knowledge of the care needed of patients and clients across the life-span and that they be able to function as members of the health care team. In recent years there has been an increased emphasis on the appropriate care of the geriatric client on the licensing exams for health care professionals. The Institute of Medicine recommended that comprehensive geriatric education be integrated though the curricula in health profession schools.[21]

Academic programs in the health sciences have chosen a variety of mechanisms to ensure that graduates are prepared to care for the aging population. Many programs integrate the aging process and associated care issues into the didactic courses in the basic and clinical sciences, while others use the clinical experiences as the mechanism to expose the students to the specifics of geriatric care. The teaching nursing home concept has been a successful strategy for educating health care professionals in interdisciplinary geriatric care.

The lack of an adequate number of faculty and clinician role models prepared in the academic area of geriatric clinical care has been cited as the main reason for schools integrating content as opposed to offering separate courses.[22] Required geriatric rotations for residency programs in internal medicine and primary care have been mandated by the Board of Internal Medicine and Family Practice as well as required geriatric client care for family nurse practitioner programs by the American Nurses Credentialing Center.

While the competencies for graduates of health care professions include the ability to function as a member of the health care team, there are no mandates from the accrediting agencies to require interdisciplinary education in the curriculum.

Only 13 medical schools require specific geriatric courses or clinical rotations.[23] Similar statistics are not available for nursing and social work. Fields, et. al.[24] found that students who had required courses and clinical rotations in geriatrics had an increased knowledge of geriatrics and improved attitude concerning the elderly.

Some programs in nursing, medicine, and social work structure the clinical experiences for the students to be able to participate in health care teams. The accreditation requirements for Geriatric Medicine Fellowship programs include a mandate for training in an interdisciplinary team. The Bureau of Health Professions in the Health Resources and Services Administration mandates interdisciplinary approaches in the Geriatric Education Centers, Geriatric Medicine and Dentistry Fellowship programs and in the interdisciplinary rural health training grants.

Recent literature in health professions education has reported an increased number of interdisciplinary educational efforts for students, particularly in the areas of child abuse, oncology and geriatrics. However, the majority of health professional education programs do not have structured required interdisciplinary educational experiences or content.

Vision for the Future

The vision for interdisciplinary education is broad for both education and practice. This vision is predicated on sound reasoning and practical considerations as outlined in the sections above.

The vision for the future is that every older person will have access to appropriate interdisciplinary health care and that every health care organization and setting providing care to older adults will have an interdisciplinary geriatric service or program with financial support for interdisciplinary practice. This does not imply that every older person would be seen by an interdisciplinary team. It does mean, however, that every institution will have an interdisciplinary team which will evaluate those individuals whose needs dictate a comprehensive assessment approach. At a minimum, the core interdisciplinary team will include a physician, a nurse, and a social worker. While ongoing participation by representatives of other disciplines is preferable, this is not always feasible, and, under these circumstances, representatives of other disciplines will be included as needed. All older people will have access to an array of health professionals as determined by an appropriate screening procedure.

Every health professional who cares for older individuals will understand the principles for interdisciplinary interaction and when it is appropriate to convene an interdisciplinary team. Interdisciplinary education will be a core component of all health professional education programs and every health care professional will have the opportunity to participate in an interdisciplinary geriatric service. There will be a body of research available regarding interdisciplinary education and practice in geriatrics. Every academic health center will have a unique position of leadership in interdisciplinary geriatric education, research and practice designated at a level above the department and college, such as Vice-President or Associate Vice-President. Realizing this vision requires a comprehensive approach to the curriculum in each of the health professions.

Interdisciplinary Geriatric Education Curriculum

Interdisciplinary geriatric education will be presented as a continuum from basic to advanced concepts and principles; from undergraduate to graduate levels (or pre-clinical to clinical levels) of education and presented in different formats in both academic and clinical settings. This educational approach encourages interdisciplinary education to be offered early in the course of a student's academic career to acquaint him/her with the benefits of interdisciplinary assessment and treatment. Initially, this may entail an individual faculty member from a single discipline describing the operation and outcomes of health care teams to students having the same major in college. Later, the students from a single discipline may be exposed to faculty from multiple disciplines or professions to gain an understanding of the knowledge and skills that each possess. It is critical that students become grounded in the knowledge, skills, approaches and values of their selected discipline or profession before they concentrate on the processes and uniqueness of team functioning and outcomes. Eventually, the goal is to have students from multiple disciplines being taught didactically in the classroom by multiple faculty and in a clinical setting by an interdisciplinary clinical geriatric team (see Figure 7.1).

The issues to be addressed in the education of interdisciplinary geriatric teams are: (1) how best to move from basic to advanced concepts and principles of interdisciplinary education and geriatrics and gerontology; (2) how to assist the student, to be grounded in their own profession/discipline and from there to gain an understanding and appreciation for the knowledge and skills of other professions; (3) how and when to combine the academic curriculum with the appropriate clinical curriculum in a complementary way, (4) how and when to combine age-specific content with interdisciplinary concepts and principles that are critical to providing appropriate, effective and efficient geriatric care.

The goal of the proposed curriculum is to bring both students and faculty from multiple disciplines together. Concepts and principles of team functioning in geriatrics will be presented and discussed within clinical settings.

Students will first learn the approach, values, knowledge and skills associated with their field before they participate with students from other disciplines to focus interdisciplinary care. Each step towards building understanding and cooperation among the professions will have benefits for clinical practice even if the total curriculum model in Figure 7.1 is not achieved.

The proposed interdisciplinary geriatric curriculum consists of: (1) the principles that govern the functioning of groups; (2) the concepts that deal with processing of group interactions and; (3) the content and context variables that must be dealt with in the care of geriatric patients. The following are the core principles, skills and topics that are necessary.

1. Principles of Teamwork:
   A. Mission, values, goals and objectives
   B. Definitions
   C. Leadership
   D. Basic information about management of well elderly and care of frail elderly
   E. Evaluation

2. Group Process and Team Skills:
   A. Interpersonal communication
   B. Role negotiation
   C. Conflict management
   D. Problem solving
   E. Decision making

3. Selected Topics:
   A. Competency-basic to advanced
   B. Professional role performance
   C. Terminology
   D. Ethics, economic issues, availability and access of health care
   E. Cultural diversity
   F. Health care delivery systems and case management
   G. Health outcomes and evaluations.

The strength of this curriculum is its foundation in both the classroom and clinical education. It allows students to develop knowledge and skills over time and apply them in increasingly complex environments.

Governing Principles

For a group of faculty, students or clinicians to work together towards a common set of goals and objectives, a mission and values statement must be established through consensus. The team's mission statement and the needs of its patient population will determine which disciplines are required on the team. The value of team work, the contribution of individual members, the values of the team and its members in affecting the team process and team problem-solving distinguish an interdisciplinary team from a multi-disciplinary team (see definitions, page 17).

Leadership of the team is based on expertise rather than position or authority. There are many opportunities for leadership on teams; there are the tasks to be completed, group processes to be facilitated and professional responsibilities to be carried out.

Processing Concepts

To problem-solve in an effective and efficient manner requires that each member of the team learn to communicate effectively with people who operate from different perspectives. Some individuals base decisions more on logic: what are the consequences of each possible solution; some on feelings: how will other people react to the decision; some on intuition: what are the implications beyond the facts; and some on sensing: what is currently being done and what are we working toward. The key to problem solving is recognizing all these perspectives.

Interpersonal communication skills include feedback, role negotiation, conflict analysis and resolution, interactive problem formulation and creative problem solving, along with evaluating team functioning and outcomes. These concepts, processes and skills must first be taught in the classroom and then applied in a clinical setting and discussed until they become enacted behaviors of each professional in relation to the other professional(s) with whom they work. Learning the language, jargon, metaphors, norms, values and culture of a team is critical to becoming an integral member of the team. It takes time and effort and will move faster if there is a clinical commonality with the team.

Selected Topics

There is a wide range of topics relevant to the care of older populations. Of particular concern to those who practice in interdisciplinary teams are the following:

Figure 7.1 Interdisciplinary Education in Academic and Clinical Settings

LEVEL OF EDUCATION	STUDENTS	FACULTY	FORMAT/ SETTING	CURRICULUM
Basic	students from single discipline	faculty from single discipline	didactic/ classroom	benefits of team assessments & treatments, terminology of gerontology & geriatrics
Basic	students from single discipline	faculty from multiple disciplines	didactic/ classroom	role of each profession in management of the well elderly along with care of the frail elderly, introductory team work skills, topics under Teamwork, #1, p.13
Basic	students from multiple disciplines	faculty from single disciplines and/or multiple disciplines	didactic classroom & clinical practicum/variety of clinical cases	team assessments & charting of geriatric cases
Advanced	students from single discipline	faculty from multiple disci-plines & clinical geriatric teams	case & patient based-problem solving/classroom & clinic	leadership, governing principles, communica-tion skills, processing, outcomes, evaluation, and combining of information from multiple professions
Advanced	students from multiple disciplines	faculty from single and/or multiple disci-plines/clinical geriatric teams	patient based-variety of clinical settings	interdisciplinary teaming to assess, treat and follow-up patients

Each professional needs to reach levels of competence in critical skills which are indicators of quality of care. Competencies in both basic and advanced knowledge and skills in each discipline need to be identified, taught in the curriculum and tested to ensure that graduates of programs and employees in continuing education programs have acquired and incorporated these competencies into their professional behaviors.

To provide quality care will require an understanding of the role of others in the health care system and how working together will produce better care. An understanding of the terminology used by each profession and their approach to and treatment of the patient will help to move the group of clinicians from a multidisciplinary to an interdisciplinary team. With an assertive team approach each professional will be able to provide optimum care within the limits of his/her own expertise.

The ethics of providing certain levels of care, economic constraints and the availability of and access to a continuum of health care present major challenges to health care professionals. Yet, answers to these challenges will come through discussion and experience in the classroom and in the clinical setting.

Diversity is complex and multifaceted. It encompasses differences, heterogeneity and distinctive sub-populations. Age-specific differences, race and ethnic makeup, levels of income and education, family support systems, beliefs and values impact access to services, equitable distribution of scarce resources and financing of benefits and delivery of care. Both professionals and the health care systems need to respond respectfully and effectively to patients, caregivers and family members in ways that affirm their human worth and preserves their dignity.

The various health care settings in which the elderly are assessed, treated and may reside determine to a great extent the type and quality of care that will be provided. Both the formal support system (local, state and national agencies) and the informal support system (family, neighbors, friends, etc.) play a major part in the maintenance and care of elderly people. Case management for clients with multiple systems needs requires a high level of understanding of the broader state and national programs and commitment to social advocacy for the health care of the clients and their caregivers. Students should be required to learn about resources available to older people, their caregivers and family members. Clinical education should include experiences based in the community.

Understanding the role of evaluation as it can be practically applied in examining how care is provided and the outcome of that care is an important component of every student's education. Evaluation and the assurance of quality care are linked and must be addressed throughout the student's experience.

Summary

The nation must have practitioners with expanded abilities and new attitudes to meet society's evolving health care needs and the needs of the growing geriatric population. The educational community is being challenged to educate a workforce that is not only competent and competitive, but also able to think critically and solve yet to be identified problems. Interdisciplinary education both in the classroom and clinical setting is an approach which will prepare students willing to work together to solve challenges in the health care arena of tomorrow.

RECOMMENDATIONS

Education

1. Interdisciplinary geriatric education will be a core requirement for every student entering a health profession.

Rationale

Approximately 60% of all users of health care services are over the age of 65 which means that almost every health care professional becomes involved with caring for older persons whether in private practice, acute care, long term care in the community or in a nursing home. Older persons generally present with chronic, long term health problems and a multitude of interrelated social and environmental issues, requiring the combined skills and knowledge of numerous disciplines (at a minimum medicine, nursing and social work). Furthermore, students in the health professions are often educated in environments which limit interaction with students from other disciplines. They learn in isolation from one another and yet are expected to work as an effective member of a health care team when they enter the workplace.

Action Required

1) The Bureau of Health Professions and the U.S. Department of Veterans Affairs will convene to develop a consensus statement on interdisciplinary geriatric education.
2) Accrediting bodies for each of the health professions and the professional associations will require the inclusion of interdisciplinary geriatric content in the curricula. This will include both didactic content to be presented in the classroom and practice oriented content to be experienced in the practice/clinical setting.
3) State licensing agencies will include questions pertaining to interdisciplinary geriatric care in the licensing examinations.
4) Academic institutions and health profession schools will develop collaborative interdisciplinary geriatric models for education of these students.

Responsible Agents

1) The Bureau of Health Professions and directors of interdisciplinary programs of the U. Department of Veterans Affairs.
2) Accrediting bodies for health care professions.
3) State licensing agencies.
4) The administrators and deans of undergraduate, graduate and post-graduate academic institutions and schools.

Expected Outcomes

1) Within 2 years a consensus document on interdisciplinary geriatric education will be submitted to all accrediting bodies of all health and associated health professions.
2) Within 3 years, 25% of the accrediting bodies will have included interdisciplinary geriatric content as a curricular requirement; within 5 years, 50% of the accrediting bodies will have reached this goal.
3) Two thirds of the states will include questions on interdisciplinary geriatric care in their licensing examinations within 5 years.
4) Academic institutions and health profession schools will respond in concert with the accrediting bodies, providing interdisciplinary geriatric education as a core requirement to their students. Five percent of the institutions and schools will offer this core before the requirements take effect, the remaining 95% will comply with the requirement beginning with the first academic year after the issuance of the requirements.

2. Health care professionals will receive continuing education concerning interdisciplinary geriatric care.

Rationale

Health care professionals currently working with older persons have rarely received any formal education regarding interdisciplinary care and yet are expected to work collaboratively and function as interdisciplinary team members. Continuing educational opportunities both within the clinical setting and the classroom can compensate for this gap in the educational preparation of health professionals.

Action Required

1) Implementation of continuing education seminars, workshops and courses on interdisciplinary geriatric care by academic institutions.
2) Inclusion of interdisciplinary geriatric care as content in seminars/workshops sponsored by professional membership organizations for continuing education units, (CEUs).
3) Inclusion of interdisciplinary geriatric care as part of in-staff training within clinical settings i.e., grand rounds, lunch time meetings, etc.

Responsible Agents

1) Geriatric and gerontology centers within academic institutions, Geriatric Education Centers, (GECs).
2) Professional membership organizations including but not limited to American Medical Association (AMA), American Osteopathic Association (AOA), American Nursing Association (ANA), the Council on Social Work Education (CSWE), American Geriatrics Society (AGS), Gerontological Society of America (GSA), and the Association for Gerontology in Higher Education (AGHE).
3) Education directors and training coordinators of membership organizations, acute care facilities, nursing homes, and community clinics.

Expected Outcomes

1) A minimum of ten additional GECs and five other geriatric/gerontology centers will offer interdisciplinary geriatric education to health care professionals within 3 years.
2) Five professional membership organizations will offer interdisciplinary geriatric care seminars to their membership for continuing education credit within 3 years.
3) The number of clinical staff training programs offered, both by membership organizations and health care facilities that include content on interdisciplinary geriatric care will double within 3 years and double again by the end of the century.

3. All health professional schools designate one or more persons as interdisciplinary geriatric educator(s).

Rationale

Interdisciplinary geriatric education is not viewed as the responsibility of a specific school or department and unless there is a funded mandate, such as that within the U.S. Department of Veterans Affairs or Geriatric Education Centers interdisciplinary geriatric education may be overlooked. This tendency can be countered by the identification of one or more persons to take responsibility for interdisciplinary education. An academic institution that identifies a person at the administrative, coordinating level and individuals within the various health professions schools to take responsibility for this area, creates a network of interested faculty with administrative support for interdisciplinary activities.

Action Required

1) Academic institutions providing professional health care education at the undergraduate, graduate and post-graduate levels will designate an individual at the administrative, organizational level and one or more faculty within each health care school or department to assume leadership for interdisciplinary geriatric education.
2) Membership organizations and professional education bodies related to the health professions will issue advisory memorandums to health care schools recommending the designation of faculty to assume leadership for interdisciplinary geriatric education.
3) The Bureau of Health Professions (BHPr) of the federal government with foundation support will develop and disseminate recommendations to health care schools concerning the development of faculty leadership in interdisciplinary geriatric education.

Responsible Agents

1) Presidents, Provosts, and administrators of academic institutions and Deans and Chairs of health profession schools and departments within these institutions.
2) Membership organizations and professional educational bodies related to health care.
3) Bureau of Health Professions in partnership with interested foundations, e.g., the Pew Foundation, Hartford Foundation.

Expected Outcomes

1) A minimum of five academic institutions will designate administrators and faculty to be responsible for interdisciplinary geriatric education within three years.
2) A minimum of five membership organizations and professional education bodies will recommend the designation of faculty to be responsible for interdisciplinary education, also within 3 years.
3) A partnership between the Bureau of Health Professions and foundations will develop and disseminate detailed recommendations within 2 years.

4. Funding will be available for faculty development to build a cadre of faculty and clinicians in interdisciplinary geriatric teamwork.

Rationale

Most health and social service professionals lack a knowledge and experiential base in interdisciplinary functioning and geriatrics. While several reports (NIA, IOM, AoA, AGHE) have identified the lack of prepared professionals in geriatrics, the professional organizations, institutions of higher education and the private practice fields have not been able to meet the targeted number of geriatric clinicians or graduates. In addition, most curriculum guides or standards of practice do not detail what is required for interdisciplinary geriatric teamwork. Yet, many of the reports speak to critical provider knowledge and skills.

Actions Required

1) The Bureau of Health Professions will take the lead in coordinating several initiatives across government agencies and private foundations to provide funding for faculty released time and faculty scholarships to allow faculty to participate in a study experience for 12 months (either half or full time).
2) New, junior and mid-career level faculty will be trained in interdisciplinary geriatric team concepts and experience working in teams. At the completion of the experience, faculty will be required to make a written report that will detail an interdisciplinary education process experience with expected

outcomes that will be implemented at their institution of higher education.

Responsible Agents

1) The Bureau of Health Professions, the Department of Veterans Affairs and Geriatric Education Centers together with professional associations (AMA, AOA, ANA, CSWE, etc.) will initiate programs for faculty development in interdisciplinary geriatric education.
2) Academic institutions will recruit new faculty or identify already employed faculty who desire further training in interdisciplinary geriatric education.

Expected Outcomes

1) The federal agencies and professional associations will have established 3 faculty scholarships within 2 years, 6 in 3 years and 12 by the turn of the century.
2) Academic institutions will submit 12 applications for faculty scholarships within 2 years, 24 within 3 years and 36 by the end of 5 years.

5. Development of interdisciplinary education materials using electronic technologies.

Rationale

In order to teach current faculty, clinical preceptors and students associated with colleges and universities across the nation, interdisciplinary education materials will be produced by electronic means. Experts in interdisciplinary geriatric education will develop educational materials designed for electronic delivery to a national audience so that faculty in urban, rural and frontier geographic areas can participate. The long-distance education technology, i.e., computer-assisted instruction, teleconferencing, interactive video, library data base access systems, interactive and multimedia programming is available but funding is required to develop the materials.

Actions Required

1) Federal, state and local government agencies will issue directives supportive of the development of electronically delivered education.
2) Private foundations, government agencies and professional and educational organizations will fund the development and delivery of these education packages.
3) Academic faculty and professionals in health care facilities will apply for development funds.

Responsible Agents

1) Bureau of Health Professions, The Learning Center for Interactive Technology of the Education Technology Branch of the Lister Hill National Center for Biomedical Communication, Institute on Medicine, National Institute on Aging, U.S. Department of Education and State Departments of Education.
2) National, State and local foundations along with professional educational associations.
3) University Medical and Nursing Informatics Department faculty, Sigma Theta Tau National Nursing Library staff, professionals and educators in health care facilities.

Expected Outcomes

1) There will be five new grant and scholarship programs funded by government agencies for faculty to develop interdisciplinary education materials by electronic means within two years. 2) Private foundations, professional organizations and government agencies will sponsor 5 career development and 5 program development projects within 2 years.

3) Ten development project grants will be awarded to academic institutions and professionals at health care facilities.

6. Interdisciplinary academic activities of faculty will be recognized as meritorious in considerations for promotion and tenure.

Rationale

Because of its own nature, interdisciplinary geriatric education is not viewed as the responsibility of any one discipline. Any interdisciplinary educational activities undertaken by a faculty person are often judged negatively as taking time away from the specific discipline or, at best, overlooked as being valueless to the department or school. Hence, interdisciplinary academic activities—curriculum development, team teaching, research, authorship of articles/ books on the subject—are not considered achievements that rate promotion or tenure. As a result, interested faculty may minimize their involvement and leadership regarding interdisciplinary geriatric education as little reward is gained and there may even be penalties within the job setting.

Action Required

1) Professional education bodies in the health care disciplines will issue directives encouraging the recognition of interdisciplinary academic activities as meritorious.
2) Administrative officers will revise guidelines and protocols for promotion and tenure to include interdisciplinary academic activities as credible academic pursuits.

Responsible Agents

1) Professional education bodies of each health care discipline e.g., Association of College Professors (ACP), Licensed College of Medical Examiners (LCME), American Osteopathic Association (AOA), American Association of Colleges of Nursing (AACN), Council of Social Work Education (CSWE), etc. 2) Administrative officers of academic institutions, Deans and Department Chairs of health profession schools.

Expected Outcomes

1) A minimum of six of the professional educational bodies representing the health disciplines will prepare statements and issue directives to their memberships in support of interdisciplinary academic activities in tenure and promotion decisions within 3 years.
2) One third of all academic institutions, schools and departments related to health care in the U.S. will issue revised guidelines for promotion and tenure to include interdisciplinary academic activities, within 5 years.

7. Chairs in interdisciplinary geriatric health care will be established in academic institutions.

Rationale

Interdisciplinary geriatric education is, by its nature, a cross-cutting modality and no one school or department in academia is viewed as owning interdisciplinary geriatric education as a field or endeavor. This often leaves the modality without academic leadership. The creation of chairs, endowed by public and/or private funds will establish a focus and reinforce the credibility of interdisciplinary geriatric education. The chairs will further promote curricula, research and practice in interdisciplinary geriatric health care.

Action Required

Endowment monies will be donated to academic institutions specifically for the underwriting of chairs in interdisciplinary geriatric health studies.

Responsible Agents

Foundations indicating interest in geriatric education e.g., the Pew, Hartford, Robert Wood Johnson, and Kellog Foundations; private corporate entities such as pharmaceutical companies and health networks.

Expected Outcomes

Within 2 years, three endowed chairs in interdisciplinary geriatric health care will be created and, by the end of the century, eight endowed chairs will be in existence.

Practice

8. Interdisciplinary geriatric teams will be the predominant model for delivering health care services to frail elderly persons and will include at a minimum, professionals from medicine, nursing and social work.

Rationale

The complex health care needs of frail elderly persons demand knowledge, skills, and expertise that no one discipline can adequately provide alone. The minimum requirement of medicine, nursing and social work representation on the team does not limit the team to these three disciplines. However, it is generally not feasible to have all disciplines represented at all times and participation in the interdisciplinary team may fluctuate, being largely determined by the facts of each individual case. Not only are clients needs becoming more complex, but so are the systems in which care is provided. Systems of care for the frail elderly are multidimensional; spanning acute care, long term care and community based care. It is beyond the scope of any one discipline to have the knowledge and expertise necessary to function at these many different levels. A team of health professionals, working together to collaborate in the planning and implementation of health care interventions are also more able to provide the comprehensive set of services necessary to address complex needs of populations with multiple interacting problems. Furthermore, it is necessary that health professionals be able to coordinate services across a continuum of care which is often fragmented and confusing. Through working together as a team, these professionals are better able to use resources appropriately to provide needed services.

Action Required

1) Accrediting bodies will include standards requiring interdisciplinary teams of health professionals based on the particular needs of the population served.
2) Comprehensive academic health science centers will develop teams in all practice settings comprised of a physician or mid-level practitioner, (physician assistant, nurse practitioner), nurse and social worker at a minimum.
3) Facility licensing bodies will require care delivered by an interdisciplinary team of health professionals composed of physician or mid-level practitioner, (physician assistant, nurse practitioner), nurse and social worker at a minimum.

Responsible Agents

1) Joint Commission for Accreditation of Healthcare Organizations (JCAHO), other accrediting bodies of clinical practice sites and state licensing bodies.
2) Association of Academic Health Science Centers (AAHSC).
3) State licensing bodies.

Expected Outcomes

1–3) All organizations providing services to complex older adults will have interdisciplinary teams in place within the next 5 years.

9. Mentors, preceptors and faculty will have educational opportunities to become experts in interdisciplinary team practice in geriatrics.

Rationale

While there is a need to develop faculty who will teach interdisciplinary geriatrics in the context of a didactic classroom there is a parallel need to develop faculty who will teach interdisciplinary geriatrics in clinical settings. When students are able to take classroom-based education, observe its application in the practice setting, and practice the application of the interdisciplinary team approach under the supervision of interdisciplinary prepared clinicians, the likelihood of instilling the desired practice behaviors is greatly increased.

Actions Required

1) Professional associations will require competency in interdisciplinary geriatric practice.
2) Standards of practice in geriatric care will include assessment and treatment by geriatric practice teams where indicated by disease or level of frailty.
3) Geriatric practice teams need to be operational in public and private medical centers, nursing homes, home care agencies and clinics.
4) Interdisciplinary geriatric teams will accept the teaching function as part of their clinical responsibilities.

Responsible Agents

1) Professional associations: AMA, AOA, ANA, NASW.
2) Professional association committees charged with writing and revising standards of practice.
3) Public and private health care facilities.
4) Members of geriatric health care teams.

Expected Outcomes

1) The Professional associations (at a minimum medicine, nursing and social work) will establish competency statements on interdisciplinary geriatric practice within 2 years.
2) Standards of practice for interdisciplinary geriatric care will be written within 3 years.
3) At least 50% of health care facilities in each state will have interdisciplinary geriatric health care teams operating within 4 years.
4) At least 50% of the interdisciplinary geriatric health care teams will include students within 4 years.

10. Definitions for interdisciplinary team practice will be developed and standards and guidelines for implementation across the continuum of care will be established.

Rationale

Although the word "team" is often used to describe the model by which care is delivered to frail older adults, there is little understanding about the meaning of interdisciplinary teamwork and how it should be implemented. Thus, there is little consistency in the approach to providing care by a team and, because no two teams are alike, it is difficult to describe what in fact is happening or to make generalizations about the actual effects of team care.

Action Required

1) Develop standards and guidelines for the implementation of interdisciplinary health

care teams across the continuum of services provided for older adults.
2) Develop continuing education activities concerning team delivery of care and how to implement it.
3) Develop demonstration programs which serve as model sites for training and delivery of interdisciplinary team care.

Responsible Agents

Agency for Health Care Policy and Research (AHCPR), The Bureau of Health Professions' Geriatric Education Centers (GEC's), in collaboration with the VA Interdisciplinary Team Training Program and the VA GRECC's.

Expected Outcomes

1) Within 3 years a set of standards would be made available by AHCPR for use by all organizations providing services to older adults. 2) A meeting will be held to develop a consensus statement about interdisciplinary geriatric teams within the next 2 years. 3) Funding will be available to support five demonstration programs within 5 years.

11. A payment/reimbursement mechanism will be implemented for services provided by the interdisciplinary geriatric team.

Rationale

Under current health care reimbursement systems there is no provision for services rendered by an interdisciplinary team of professionals. Without financial incentive there is little reason to educate health care professionals to work in interdisciplinary geriatric teams. Under traditional fee-for-service, fees are set for individual health professionals, with no incentives for interdisciplinary care. The interdisciplinary team approach may appear to take additional time initially, but in the long-term brings savings to the system by better coordinated care at the most appropriate level. There must be provision to cover the interdisciplinary aspects of care taking into account numbers of patients served, acuity level of patients, and outcomes of care.

Action Required

1) The development of funding mechanisms through Medicare and Medicaid to include interdisciplinary team care based on the acuity level of the patient and the intensity of team resources required.
2) Insurance coverage reflecting this funding mechanism.
3) Incorporation of funding for interdisciplinary collaboration in managed care.

Responsible Agents

1) Health Care Financing Administration (HCFA).
2) Health Insurance companies.
3) Managed care organizations.

Expected Outcomes:

1–3) Funding mechanisms to cover interdisciplinary team care will be developed and piloted in 2 years and implemented on a national level in 5 years.

Research

12. An Interdisciplinary Geriatric Research Fellowship will be developed and funded.

Rationale

Currently there are no fellowships that develop research leadership with a focus on interdisciplinary geriatric practice or education. The specific nuances in methodology and analysis that are required to assess outcomes of interdisciplinary education and practice need to be identified and taught to other researchers. Without specific research attention to this field, the questions regarding the efficacy of interdisciplinary education and practice will continue. Both the Department of Veterans Affairs and the Bureau of Health Professions have sustained commitments to interdisciplinary geriatric education and practice. Both organizations have fellowship programs and the VA funds Geriatric Research, Education and Clinical Centers and Interdisciplinary Team Training Programs which would provide research sites for the fellows.

Action Required

Initiate and fund a new fellowship in Interdisciplinary Geriatric Research.

Responsible Agents

Department of Veterans Affairs jointly with the Bureau of Health Professions.

Expected Outcomes

The first fellowship position designated as Interdisciplinary Geriatric Research and focused on assessing education and practice outcomes will be announced within 3 years.

13. Existing geriatric/gerontology focused fellowships in nursing, medicine, social work, dentistry, psychology, psychiatry, etc. will include education and experience in research in interdisciplinary geriatric education and practice.

Rationale

In order for interdisciplinary geriatric care to become fully integrated into professional health training, it is necessary to develop educators and clinicians to act as mentors and teachers. One means of developing this leadership is to provide opportunities for doctoral and post-doctoral students to immerse themselves in the content area and acquire expertise. Existing fellowship programs in geriatrics/gerontology provide educational opportunities to develop leaders with this research expertise. By strengthening the interdisciplinary curriculum component in the existing fellowship programs a cadre of role models and leaders in interdisciplinary geriatric care will be created.

Action Required

Funds will be offered to support, within existing geriatric/gerontology fellowship programs, the development of interdisciplinary curriculum models and experiences which focus on research methodologies and analyses which study interdisciplinary geriatric teams and their impact on patient care.

Responsible Agents

Foundations (e.g., Hartford, Pew, etc.), professional membership organizations (e.g., Gerontological Society of America, American Nursing Association, etc.), academic institutions, U.S. Department of Health and Human Services, Veterans Affairs, and the host settings for the fellowships, i.e., VA Medical Centers, Hospitals, long-term care facilities.

Expected Outcomes

The interdisciplinary research curricular model will be included in fellowships in medicine, nursing and social work within the first 3 years and another three fellowships within another 2 years.

14. Research will be directed towards the evaluation of interdisciplinary geriatric education and practice outcomes.

Rationale

There is a dearth of rigorous scientific literature about outcomes of interdisciplinary approaches to geriatric team education and practice. There are few comparative studies which assess differences in educational or patient outcomes. Thus, there is concern that much of what is known about teams is based on myth, assumption, misinformation, or failure to even consider who provides the care and how it is provided. Yet, those who work in teams advocate that education about interdisciplinary team skills is not only critical but results in better patient outcomes.

Actions Required

1) Funding will be made available to support research efforts focused on the delivery of geriatric care by an interdisciplinary team. The research will address educational outcomes, team processing and outcomes of team care.
2) Strategies for developing approaches to conduct health services research on interdisciplinary teams need to be developed.

Responsible Agents

1) The National Institute on Aging, National Science Foundation, The U.S. Department of Veterans Affairs, and the Bureau of Health Professions will provide grants for research on educational and patient outcomes associated with interdisciplinary education and practice.
2) The fellowship programs described in the research recommendations #1 and #2 above will provide leadership and expertise in devising research strategies.

Expected Outcomes

1) Two grants for research will be made available within 3 years and an additional two grants will be available within another 2 years.
2) Research strategies to be used in studying the results of interdisciplinary education and practice will be included in the grant announcements that are issued within the 3-year and additional 2-year periods.

REFERENCES

1. Luszki M. 1958 Interdisciplinary team research methods and problems. NY, National Training Laboratories as cited in Given B and Simmons S. The interdisciplinary health care team: Fact or fiction?" Nursing Forum 1977; 16 165–184.
2. Baldwin DC, Tsukuda RAW. Interdisciplinary teams, Chap 30. In Cassel, C, Walsh, JR ed. Fundamentals of Geriatric Medicine. New York: Springer, 1984.
3. Clark PG; Spence D Sheehan JL. A service learning model for interdisciplinary teamwork in health and aging. Gerontology and Geriatrics Education, Vol. 6, (4) Summer 1986.
4. Solomon D, Steel K, Williams TF, Brown AS, Brummel-Smith K, Buirgess L, D'Agostino RB, Goidschmidt JW, Halter JB, Hazzard WR, Jahnigen DW, Phelps C, Raskind M, Schrier RW, Sox HC, Williams SV, Wykle M. National Institutes of health consensus development conference statement: geriatric assessment methods for clinical decision making. J Am Ger Soc 1988; 36:342–347.
5. Rubenstein LZ, Josephson KR, Wieland GD, English PA, Sayre JA, Kane RL. Effectiveness of a geriatric evaluation unit: a randomized trial. N Engl J Med 1984; 311:1664–70.
6. Williams ME, Williams TF, Zimmer JG, Hall WJ, Podgorski CA. How does the team approach to outpatient geriatric evaluation compare with traditional care: a report of a randomized controlled trial. J Am Ger Soc 1987; 35:1071–1078.
7. Rubenstein LV, Calkins DR, Young RT, Cleary PD, Fink A, Kosecoff J, Jette AM, Davies AR, Delhanco TL, Brook RH. Improving patient function: a randomized trial of functional disability screening. Ann

Intern Med 1989; 111:836–842.
8. Calkins DR, Rubenstein LV, Cleary PD, Davies AR, Jette AM, Fink A, Koseoff J, Young RT, Brook RH, Delbanco TL. Functional disability screening of ambulatory patients: A randomized controlled trial in a hospital-based group practice. J Gen Intern Med 1994; 9:590–592.
9. Rubenstein LZ, Stuck AE, Siu AL, Wieland D. Impacts of geriatric evaluation and management programs on defined outcomes: overview of the evidence. J Am Ger Soc 1991; 398:88–168.
10. Bass B. Team productivity and individual member competence. Small Group Behavior 1980; 11:431–504.
11. Campion E, Jette A, Berman B. An interdisciplinary geriatric consultation service: A controlled trial. J. Am Geriatr Soc 1983; 31(12):792–296.
12. Zimmer J, Groth-Juncker A, McCusker J. A randomized controlled study of a home health care team. Am J Pub Health 1985; 75:134–141.
13. Poulin J, Walter C, Walker J. Interdisicplinary team membership: A survey of gerontological social workers. J Gero Soc Work 1994; 22(1/2): 93–107.
14. Mellor J. The interdisciplinary nature of social work practice in geriatric health care settings. Doctoral dissertation, City University of New York, 1994.
15. Wise, H, Beckhard, R, Rubin, I, Kyte, A. (eds). Making health teams work. Cambridge, MA: Ballinger Publishing Co. 1974.
16. Parker,AW. The team approach to primary health care, Berkeley, University of California. 1972.
17. Faulkner A. Interdisciplinary health care teams: an educational approach to improvement of health care for the aged. Gerontology and Geriatrics Education. 1985; Vol 5, No. 3, 29–39.
18. Pew Health Professions Commission. Health America: Practitioners for 2005. San Francisco: The Pew Charitable Trust. 1991.
19. Joint Commission on Accreditation of Healthcare Organizations. The Measurement Mandate. Oakbrook Terrace, Ill: JCAHO, 1993.
20. Povar GJ. Continuous quality improvement and primary care: holding ourselves accountable. Primary Care Policy Fellow Report. 1994; 2(1):2,7–8.
21. Brooks TR. Attitudes of medical students and family practice resident toward geriatric patients. Journal of National Medical Association. 1993; 85(1):61–4.
22. Katz PR, Kunza J, Hall, N. Residency education in the nursing home: a national survey of internal medicine and family practice programs. J Gen Int Med 1992; 7(1);52–6.
23. Kowal J. Meeting geriatric physician needs: Problems facing current training activities. Shortage of health care professions caring for the elderly; Recommendation for change. Report lect Committee on Aging. Washing, DC: Comm Pub No. 1992. 102–915.
24. Fields SD, Jutagir R, Adaman RD, Tiedeiksarr R, Olsen, E. Geriatric education Part 1: Efficacy of a mandatory clinical rotation for fourth year medical students. Am Ger Soc: 409. 1992; (9):964–9, Sept.

8

Ethnogeriatrics

Neil Henderson, Melvina McCabe, Veronica J. Scott, Melissa Talamantes, Barbara W. K. Yee, and Gwen Yeo

THE STATE OF THE ART OF ETHNOGERIATRIC EDUCATION AND TRAINING

Introduction

This paper traces the developing awareness of an important and timely issue for the future of geriatric education in the U.S.—the ability of health care providers to care for the expanding population of elders from diverse backgrounds with competence and confidence. After an exploration of the need and historical development of ethnogeriatric education, the authors project their vision of what an adequate system would include in the 21st century. On the basis of this vision, policy recommendations are made to provide the basis of a stable and effective system to train future providers for the diversity they will meet in geriatric care.

The terminology in this paper reflects the current usage, which is frequently overlapping and less precise than one might desire in a strict nosology. The term "culture" refers, in short, to the way of life of a population, or part of a population. Although it is used most often with reference to different societies or national origins, it can also reflect differences by geographic regions or other subgroups within a nation. The term "race" implies physical or biological groupings of people, and "minority" is used to describe not only a numerical, but also a power disadvantage. The term "ethnic" is used heavily in this paper since it carries a somewhat broader meaning. While "ethnicity" most often identifies a difference based on culture, it is also used for groups identified by racial or religious differences. The multiethnic team of authors from several disciplines see culture as the overriding issue on which geriatric education on diversity should be focused, although racial differences and minority status need to be included.

Since much of the information on diversity of elders comes from U.S. government sources such as census data, the categories used in those sources necessarily shape the groupings around which information is summarized. For that reason the population categories of African American, American Indian/Alaska Native, Asian/Pacific Island

Table 8.1 Percent of Persons 65+ in U.S. by Race and Hispanic Origin

POPULATION	1990	2030 (Projected)
White*	86.7%	74.6%
Black*	7.9%	9.1%
American Indian/ Eskimo & Aleut*	0.3%	0.5%
Asian & Pacific Islander*	1.4%	5.0%
Hispanic Origin	3.7%	10.9%
TOTAL	**100.0%**	**100.1%**

* Not hispanic
Source: U.S. Bureau of the Census & National Institute on Aging, 1993. Racial and Ethnic Division of America's Elderly Population

American, and Hispanic American are used most often even though they may not be the most significant categories. The four categories are racial designations except "Hispanic", which is usually described as "ethnic", although all four categories include many different ethnic groups. Individuals classified as "Hispanic" can be of any race. It should be noted that in almost all sources of information individuals report their own racial or ethnic identification. To simplify the reporting in this paper the four federally designated categories are referred to as "ethnic" or "ethnic minority."

Historical Background

Need

Geriatric educators in the coming decades will face the growing challenge of preparing health care providers for the tremendous variation they will see in the ethnic background of their older patients. The ethnic minority populations of older Americans are growing even faster than the exploding population of older adults as a whole (see Table 8.1). By 2030, elders from populations classified as ethnic minority (African American, American Indian/Alaska Native, Asian/ Pacific Island American, and Hispanic American) are projected to make up one fourth of all older Americans.[1] In some states diversity of the older population is already substantial. In the nation's most populous state, California, for example, elders of color already comprise over 20% of the older population and are projected to reach 41% by 2020.[2, 3]

Both between and within each of the major ethnic categories, including those classified as white, vast differences are found in factors which affect the health and health care of older adults. Differences include patterns of health beliefs and health care utilization, health risks, patterns of interdependence with family members, ethical decision making priorities, and, in some cases, response to treatment.

Intra-category Diversity. The heterogeneity *within* the categories currently used to describe major ethnic populations in the U.S. produces considerable complexity of the subject matter in ethnogeriatrics. Diversity exists within each of the ethnic minority categories, and also within the majority category of Non-Hispanic white, who are most often labeled merely "white", or "Anglo." Although the intra-category variability may be obvious, a few examples are provided to emphasize the point.

1. More than thirty different national origins are found among the elders lumped together in the most rapidly growing designation, the "Asian/Pacific Islanders"(A/PI). The percentage of A/PI elders born outside the U.S. range from 28% for Japanese to virtually 100% for Vietnamese and Cambodian, with the large Chinese and Filipino groups estimated to be 81% and 96% respectively, and many health risks have been consistently found to vary with place of birth.[4] Even among elders labeled "Chinese", examples of diversity are evident: 1) at least four different major language groups, and English proficiency ranging from little or none to fluent even among elders who have been in the U.S. for several decades; 2) elders born in the U.S., mainland China, Taiwan, Hong Kong, and Vietnam; 3) significant proportions whose educational backgrounds vary from no years of schooling to graduate degrees; 4) some of the wealthiest and some of the poorest elders in the U.S.; 5) some who use traditional Chinese therapies and medications before, some during, and some after going to a Western medical provider, and some who never do; 6) many who live with adult children and depend on them for care if needed, and many who prefer to live independently.

2. The second most rapidly growing ethnic minority population of U.S. elders are those labeled "Hispanic." This includes those who immigrated recently as older "followers of children" to be close to adult offspring; it also includes substantial numbers whose ancestors moved into the area which is now part of the U.S. while it was still Mexico, or even before there was a Mexico, as well as elders born in the U.S. of families who have immigrated more recently. Large numbers born in Puerto Rico and Cuba are also part of this populations whose reasons for coming to the U.S. may have been dramatically different. There are currently relatively small numbers of elders from Central and South America, but in the future their number will grow as individuals who have come as political refugees grow older. Vast differences are also found in wealth, education, rural/urban residence, family size, family support, acculturation, English proficiency, and use of folk healing traditions.

3. There are over 500 identified tribal backgrounds among elders classified as "American Indian/Eskimo or Aleut." Some are living in the most remote and isolated rural, and most poverty stricken areas in the country, yet almost half are living in cities and other urban areas where the Indian Health Service benefits are much less available than on reservations. In some tribes, large proportions of elders have zero years of schooling; many other elders in the present cohort were removed as children and educated in boarding schools long distances from their parents and communities to force acculturation to the American way of life. Others were part of the forced relocation to urban areas in the 1940s and 1950s, where many are now an invisible sector of those cities. Some are strong advocates of the native Indian health

traditions in which health and spirituality are heavily linked, and others are regular participants in the Western biomedical health care system.

4. Elders in the largest category, the "Black" population, are composed of subgroups representing vastly different extremes in rural/urban, regional, educational, income, and religious backgrounds. Although most of today's older African Americans were born in the U.S., in the future there will be a growing population of "Black" elders who were born in the Caribbean or Africa and immigrated to the U.S. during young adulthood. A large proportion of the current cohort of African American elders spent their early years in the South where they experienced severe exploitation and legalized discrimination, including a segregated health care system. Those whose families lived in the north were also likely to have been objects of the widespread racial discrimination and prejudice of the early 20th century, even though it was less likely to be legally authorized as in the South.

5. While it may seem obvious, the tremendous heterogeneity among the older population classified as "white" also needs to be acknowledged. Along with the vast range of characteristics among the millions of "white" elders are many cultural and religious differences that impact on the health care interaction. "White ethnic" or Euro-American groups include elders who have recently immigrated from Russia and other European countries, as well as those whose families have lived in the U.S. for one or more generations and who have preserved their various ethnic identification in neighborhoods or other networks.

Geriatric educators have paid very little attention to the ethnic diversity of older patients until now, but it is no longer acceptable for geriatric health care providers to ignore the implications of diversity to provide good health care. Almost every interaction with an older patient and every decision a provider must make about care are affected by the cultural background of that elder, from assessment of function to prescription of medications to working with family caregivers to executing advance directives about life sustaining care.

Development of the Field of Ethnogeriatric Education

What is now generally referred to as "Ethnogeriatrics" is conceptualized as the nexus of the fields of aging, health, and ethnicity (see Figure 8.1). Cultural influences on health and health care have been recognized for several decades through the discipline of medical anthropology and, more recently, transcultural nursing. It was not until late in the 1980's, however, that its application to geriatric training began to be explored in a systematic way. Likewise, the field of gerontology (the study of aging) had included cultural diversity and minority status in the courses and textbooks relating to aging since some of the major pioneering work in the 1970s, but its application to the health care disciplines was not clearly drawn until late in the decade of the 1980's, in spite of at least some earlier recognition of its importance.[5] Jacqueline J. Jackson is usually credited with coining the term "ethnogerontology" in the late 1970s to describe the arm of gerontology that explores ethnic, racial, and minority issues. In 1987, Core Faculty members of Stanford Geriatric Education Center adapted the term "ethnogeriatrics" from Dr. Jackson's contribution to describe health care for elders from different ethnic backgrounds.

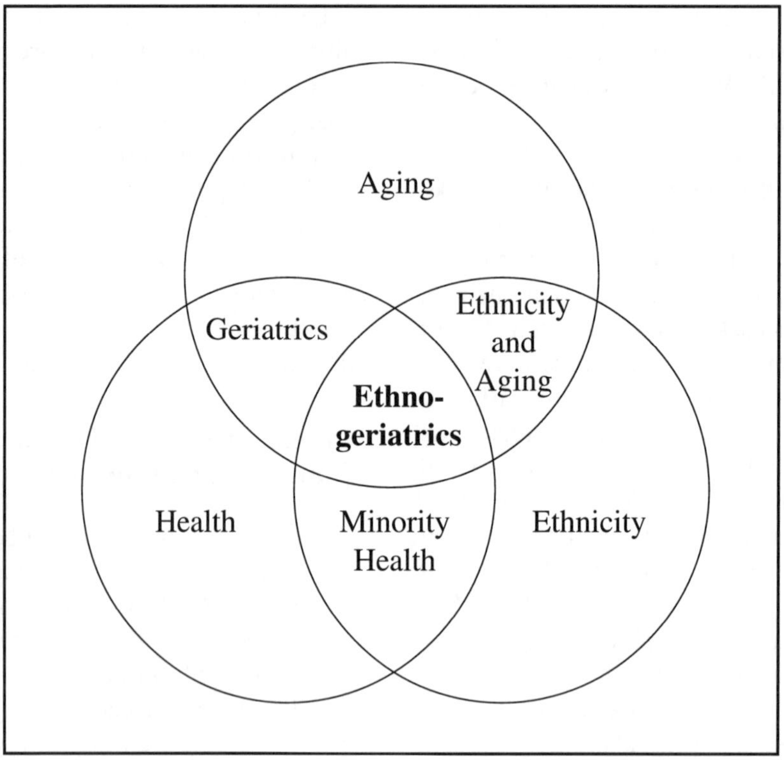

Figure 8.1

Evaluation of the Field in the 1980s. Two small efforts to assess the level of development of ethnogeriatric education were undertaken in early 1988. To explore the degree to which the health care training disciplines had included ethnogeriatrics in their curricula, Core Faculty members of the Stanford Geriatric Education Center (SGEC) reviewed 41 potential geriatric textbooks in their own disciplines. Ethnogeriatric content was identified as material that combined the three basic components of health, aging, and ethnicity. Overall, 17 of the 41 geriatric textbooks had some reference to ethnic issues, but some of the disciplines were found to be much further ahead of others in integrating ethnogeriatric concepts. All of the 3 psychology books, 71% of the 7 books in social work, 47% of the 15 gerontological nursing books, and 13% of the 15 geriatric medicine books reviewed contain ethnogeriatric material. The one geriatric textbook in occupational therapy had no ethnic content.[6]

In addition to text resources, a modest effort to assess course offerings in ethnogeriatrics was also undertaken in 1988. Listings of courses in the *National Directory of Educational Programs* published in 1987 by the Association of Gerontology in Higher Education (AGHE)[7] were reviewed for content in "ethnic" or "minority" or "cross-cultural" issues in aging . Of the 404 colleges and universities listed, 41 had a reference to ethnogerontological content, 16 of which were associated with health care training programs. A request for information was sent to the 16 programs, all on the East or

West Coast; responses were received from 8 and 4 other schools with similar courses were identified in the process. Only one course, taught in a vocational nursing program in a California community college, combined the three components of health, aging, and ethnicity. One school reported that a cultural emphasis was included throughout their nursing curriculum, some of which applied to geriatric care. The most common pattern offered a class in ethnicity and aging in anthropology or ethnic studies program for students in different fields, including health care disciplines.[5]

Funding Preferences and Grants. A major impetus for the growth of the field was the funding preferences given by the Bureau of Health Professions (BHPr) to applicants for Geriatric Education Centers (GECs) related to minority participation. Beginning with the 1987 funding cycle, preference was given to:

> *applicants from institutions that demonstrate a commitment to increased minority participation in their program or show evidence of efforts to recruit minority faculty.*[8]

In 1989, the preference was expanded to include:

> *Applications which identify minority faculty or scholars with expertise in minority aging with substantial roles in carrying out the project. [and] Applications documenting formal linkages—with predominantly minority educational institutions or health facilities to accomplish specific aspects of the project protocol (e.g. involving minority faculty, students, or practitioners, developing curricula or expanding teaching concerning minority elderly, providing trainees with experience in caring for minority elderly, etc.).*[9]

These preferences were continued through the 1991 funding cycle. In 1993 the following preference was included and continued for 1994:

> *applications that demonstrate linkages for the purpose of training educators or practitioners who serve minority or low-income elderly.*[10]

Since the GECs have been the most important federal funding mechanism for geriatric education in multiple disciplines during the last decades, and 49 universities representing almost all states and Puerto Rico have received GEC grants for 3 or more years during that time, the impact of the funding preferences have been far reaching.

In addition to BHPr funding, the development of curricula and instruction in ethnogeriatrics in the last decade has also been spurred partially by grants from the Administration on Aging (AoA) to national aging organizations, grants from National Institute on Aging and National Institute on Mental Health for research among ethnic minority elders.

Major Events and Publications. Significant milestones in the growth of ethnogeriatric education are listed below.

1. Conference: *Minority Aging: Essential Curriculum Content for Selected Health and Allied Health Professionals.* In February, 1988, a national invitational 2-day conference was sponsored by the BHPr of the Health Resources and Services Administration and the Health, Alcohol, Drug Abuse, and Mental Health Administrations of the National Institute of Mental (ADAMHA) for approximately 100 experts on health care for minority elders and geriatric educators. The conference grew out of concerns by key staff about the lack of curriculum related to minority aging in health care training. The focus was on the development of curriculum content and approaches in teaching health professionals issues that affect the health care of elders from disadvantaged minority backgrounds.

2. Book: *Minority Aging: Essential Curricula Content for Selected Health and Allied Health Professions.* The papers presented at the conference described above formed the basis of this volume edited by Dr. Mary Harper of ADAMHA and published in 1990.[11] The book contains 42 chapters which focus on: reviews of the major demographic, health status, utilization, and treatment literature on each of the four older disadvantaged minority populations; specific disease issues of importance for individual populations; research needs and gaps; and curriculum recommendations for health professions education in general and for specific disciplines.

3. Concurrent Development of Curriculum Resources and Instructional Strategies in Several GECs, 1989-1992: By spring of 1990, ethnogeriatric education was blossoming, especially through the work of GECs. A symposium on GECs at the American Society of Aging (ASA) 1990 meeting published in 1992 documented the following contributions to the field: 24 modules or other teaching units developed by 12 GECs; 13 monographs; 7 videotapes; 36 conferences featuring ethnogeriatric topics sponsored by 20 GECs; 13 centers with clinical training sites; and 3 computerized bibliographic data bases.[12]

4. Book of Course Outlines: *Teaching About Aging: Interdisciplinary and Cross-Cultural Perspectives.* In 1991 the Association for Anthropology and Gerontology (AAGE) compiled and disseminated a collection of 30 course outlines and resources from various universities dealing with aging and culture/ethnicity. While most of the courses were taught in anthropology programs, most have content on health issues, and some were taught in health disciplines.[13]

5. Teleconference: *Ethnic Diversity: Barrier or Benefit in Health Care for the Elderly?* Sponsored by Virginia Commonwealth GEC, this national teleconference in 1991 highlighted issues in geriatric health care for the four ethnic minority categories. It was seen by an audience of several thousand across the nation and included a discussion of educational as well as clinical and policy topics.

6. Publication by Gerontological Society of America (GSA): *Minority Elders: Longevity, Economics, and Health.* Using AoA funding, the Task Force on Minority Issues of GSA sponsored the development of consensus papers related to minority aging in several health-related arenas, using a broad-based process including many participants in the field of gerontology and geriatrics. The resulting 1991 publication has been widely used as reading material in aging courses in various disciplines. GSA reissued the booklet in 1994 with updates of abstracts of 71 articles recently published in *The Gerontologist* or the *Journals of Gerontology*.[14, 15]

7. Conference: *Ethnogeriatric Curriculum: What Should We Teach and How Should We Teach It?* A two-day conference in January 1992, sponsored by Stanford and Meharry GECs, San Jose State University, and Palo Alto VA Geriatric Research Educational and Clinical Center (GRECC) was attended by 94 faculty members from 11 disciplines and 16 states. Ethnogerontological specialists recommended curricular content and demonstrated experiential instructional strategies. Workgroups developed recommended ethnogeriatric curricula for six disciplines. Instructional strategies and curricular outlines are available.

Resources Currently Available

Within the past few years, recognition of need for geriatric education concerning cultural diversity and activity in the field have been increasing at a rapid rate. Both the American Geriatrics Society (AGS) and the Clinical Medicine Section of GSA have developed special activities and committees on ethnogeriatrics. The Ethnogeriatric Task Force of AGS developed a position paper on ethnogeriatrics passed by the AGS Board, and sponsored a special symposium on Ethnogeriatric Education in its annual meeting in 1994. The Association for Gerontology in Higher Education (AGHE) encourages submissions for a track in minority aging at its annual meeting, and ASA regularly features educationally related presentations on aging and minority health.

The number of publications on ethnogeriatric topics is increasing with such rapidity that they are difficult to monitor. (The Stanford GEC Bibliographic Data Base on Ethnogeriatrics has over 2300 articles catalogued, with dozens more identified each month.) The current list of "GEC Materials Related to Minority Aging"[16] includes 18 videos, 3 syllabi, 9 curricula modules, 14 book chapters, 2 training manuals, 5 literature reviews, 10 journal articles, 11 conference proceedings, 3 bibliographies, and 19 monographs or working papers. These are being used for multidisciplinary and unidisciplinary education throughout the country. Currently most GECs report some teaching activity related to minority and/or ethnicity.

Several disciplines have developed specific curricula on ethnic or minority issues that are included in geriatric textbooks or curriculum guides. These include: nursing,[17] occupational therapy,[18] optometry,[19] and social work.[20] A particularly innovative didactic and clinical curriculum in medicine was implemented by the Department of Family Practice at University of California, Irvine, using a specialized ethnogeriatric clinic.[21] A survey of public health training programs found that 20% include content on racial and ethnic minority elders;[22] a curriculum development workshop in 1992 then developed recommendations in aging and public health with resources for ethnogeriatric training which were disseminated in proceedings.[23]

Within the next year Garland Press will publish *Ethnic Diversity and the Elderly: Issues in Research and Curriculum Development*, edited by Espino, Talamantes, and Yeo, which includes ethnogeriatric curricula from programs around the country. Stanford GEC will also disseminate modules for teaching ethnogeriatric content in eight individual health professions.

Summary of the Current Status of the Field

Planning for an adequate system of geriatric education in the 21st century requires integration of the implication of the growing cultural diversity of older Americans at every level of training in all health care disciplines. A recognition of this need has motivated an increasing level of activity in the field which now must be implemented much more widely to reach all those working in geriatric education. To facilitate the ongoing process of development and integration, it is important to build on the strengths and correct the weaknesses of resources currently available.

Limitations

The current knowledge base for developing curriculum and teaching strategies to train providers to care for elders from diverse ethnic backgrounds effectively is based on input from educators from disparate disciplines and geographic areas in response to their growing perception of need. As a result, substantial variation is found in the terminology, theoretical perspectives, content, and emphases of different authors. Examples of differences in terminology include the use of "minority" or "ethnic" or "cultural" or "people of color," or some combination to denote some or all of the populations that are not "white," "majority," "Anglo," or "European American." Descriptions of individual population categories also include a number of terms by which they are identified, for example, "black" or "African American"; "Hispanic" or "Latino"; "Native American" or "American Indian" (with or without the additional designation "Alaska Native" or "Eskimo and Aleut"). Much of the ethnogeriatric literature in medicine is found in family medicine and psychiatry; to the extent that a theoretical perspective is found, it frequently is based on the work of Kleinman and his colleagues using the concept of Explanatory Models of Illness,[24] which may or not be found in the writings from other disciplinary perspectives. Much of the nursing literature comes from the work of Leininger on Transcultural Nursing.[25]

Some efforts to insert cross-cultural issues into already heavily scheduled curricula resulted in heavy reliance on stereotypes to describe cultural differences, which can result in attitudes and behavior detrimental to effective provider/patient interaction that are counterproductive to the objectives of the entire effort. All levels of depth and comprehensiveness are found in available curricular resources. Some are very narrowly focused (e.g. diabetes); others provide a basis for a broad semester-length course.[26]

Much of the research data currently available on different older ethnic populations has not been incorporated specifically into curriculum resources, and probably more importantly, many available resources on cross-cultural health care have not been specifically applied to geriatrics.

Dilemmas

It should be recognized that converting the wish to develop cultural competence among geriatric practitioners into reality introduces some difficult problems.

1. Skills overload: The expertise demanded of health care practitioners is already enormous, and it is extremely difficult to find an appropriate balance between an unrealistically high expectation of competence in behavioral/social science skills and a superficially ineffective use of cultural concepts.

2. Data overload in case management: Practitioners may be challenged to add an unrealistic amount of new cultural data to an already rich data bank.

3. Superficial use of cultural concepts: Without adequate cultural expertise, the complexities of cultural dynamics can be misinterpreted.

4. Recognition and resources for adequate trained faculty: In spite of presence of cultural content in many health science curricula, many observers rate practitioners' skills in cultural competence as inadequate. Correcting the deficit requires both a "paradigm shift" in health science training and infusion of money and political effort.

The vision of the future for ethnogeriatrics and recommendations that follow are designed to make the shortcomings and dilemmas discussed above less visible in the decades ahead.

Vision

The vision of geriatric care in the U.S. for the next century is certainly "multicolored," reflecting not only growing diversity of older patients, but also of providers of care. In an ideal future a health care system is composed of providers from diverse ethnic backgrounds who are recruited to a variety of health disciplines and taught the attitudes, knowledge, and skills necessary to provide culturally competent care. Specific components of that vision are described below.

1. Increased Diversity of Educators, Providers, and Trainees

The faculty teaching geriatrics and health care providers at all levels should represent the same diversity that is found in the population, especially at the local level. The future will hopefully see a more equal distribution of disadvantaged populations throughout the skill levels rather than the current concentration at entry level positions. Although there is no assurance that individual members of ethnic minorities have inherent ethnogeriatric expertise to care for elders from their own ethnic background, they can frequently bring insight and legitimacy to the development of a strong multiethnic climate that supports the ethnogeriatric emphasis. More importantly, ethnic minority students are likely to have important language skills and commitment to serve the population with which they are most familiar, ultimately decreasing barriers to health care access currently experienced by ethnic elders. Attention to recruitment must be followed by attention and support for career ladder movement, mentoring, promotion and tenure for faculty. Rather than token members of underrepresented populations, it is important to achieve a critical mass of cross-cultural geriatric specialists in the faculty and provider teams as well as on educational boards, advisory committees, review panels, and staff of funding agencies, in order to be able to increase the cultural competence of the educational and health services organizations.

As comprehensively described in the report "Balancing the Scales of Opportunity: Ensuring Racial and Ethnic Diversity in the Health Professions" from the Institute of Medicine (IOM),[27] it is going to be difficult to increase the pipeline of ethnic minorities in the health professions if recruitment is not begun before key educational decision points. This report suggests that educational interventions should be started before high school and continued at each stage of the student/career ladder to increase the number of ethnic minorities who eventually become providers/educators in the health arena. Targeting recruitment at each level of the pipeline could increase the small number of ethnic minority students in ethnogeriatrics currently at the doctoral level if it were implemented by multiple educational programs. The IOM report also regards enhancing diversity of health educators, providers, and trainees to be a necessary but not sufficient ingredient to improve health care for ethnic minority populations. In ethnogeriatrics, minority educators and providers as well as non-minority geriatric students, educators, and providers should be recruited and trained in diversity.

Key strategies can be learned from successful ethnic minority doctoral training programs. One exemplary model is the Minority Fellowship Program (MFP) of the

American Psychological Association (APA) funded by Substance Abuse and Mental Health Services Administration, Center for Mental Health Services, although similar programs exist through national associations of nursing. psychiatry, and sociology. Since its inception, the APA MFP has supported 730 doctoral students in psychology,[28] 54% of whom have completed their Ph.D.s; only 6% have dropped out, and the graduation rate is estimated to be 80% to 90%. Key features of the MFP are: shared responsibility with universities; 3-year awards; commitments by universities to support fellows beyond this period; and payback agreements by fellows to serve a year of service in educational settings or to underserved or seriously mentally ill populations for every year of support. Yearly tracking of student progress and potential problems assist the MFP to provide interventions on behalf of fellows such as phone contacts, mentorship support, and site visits.

Jones[29] summarizes the key qualitative features of programs committed to training ethnic minority psychologists: 1) a critical mass of 20% of ethnic minority doctoral students are needed to influence the social and intellectual environment in the departments; 2) ethnic minority faculty to provide role models for the students, and both ethnic minority and non-minority faculty sensitive to the students' needs for emotional and intellectual support; 3) courses that reflect diversity perspectives; 4) curriculum in cross-cultural research methodology and literature; 5) a practicum requiring work with multicultural populations and supervisors who can help students become more culturally responsive to the variety of clients they see; and 6) practice and discussion of culturally sensitive treatment issues.

In other programs strategies found to increase the recruitment and retention of ethnic minority trainees to serve in medically underserved areas include financial aid and flexibility of the curricular schedule to allow a part-time, extended enrollment.[30] Successful recruitment techniques for faculty and trainees in GEC programs were found to include informal networking, use of advisory committees, content with a minority focus, and "gerontologizing" minority faculty from other fields.[31]

2. Development and Implementation of Cross-Cultural Curriculum

The vision of a fully developed program in ethnogeriatric education includes a number of core components implemented in all the discipline specific geriatric curricula as well as in interdisciplinary training formats. These include but are not limited to: learning objectives, theoretical bases, course or training content, strategies for didactic and clinical instruction, and outcome evaluation measures.

Objectives and Theory. In order to guide the development of ethnogeriatric curriculum, learning objectives should be specified by outlining competencies important for health care practice with elders from diverse backgrounds specific to health profession(s) being targeted.[11] Theoretical frameworks helpful to education in cross-cultural medicine, transcultural nursing, and medical anthropology can be productively adapted to geriatrics. For example, the concept of Explanatory Models can be used as a basis to develop specific teaching techniques for understanding elders' perception of their illness and effective methods of negotiating acceptable treatment.[23, 32] Intercultural influence has been proposed as a concept to replace the more static concept of cultural diversity.[33] Models of continua of attitudes and behaviors, such as the Developmental Model of Ethnosensitivity[34] are useful constructs on which to base affective and behavioral instruction applied to geriatric care.

Content. Content for didactic and clinical teaching in cross-cultural geriatric care must be comprehensive. At the minimum, the following areas would be developed:

Intercultural Dynamics. For geriatric practitioners to provide culturally competent care, foundational principles of intercultural dynamics must be understood and practiced:

1. The concept of culture at the *community level* in which a practice is operating.
2. The concept of culture at the subgroup level within the practice community such as identification of *ethnic group culture.*
3. The concept of culture at the *individual patient* level.
4. The understanding that the *practitioner possesses a personal culture.*
5. The patient and practitioner interact under the influence of the *health care system culture*, influenced by the organization of health care delivery systems.
6. The understanding of individual culture as *multifaceted.*
   - Situational ethnicity: elder patients may reveal more or less of their "home" culture based on the nature of the social setting in which they are behaving.
   - Acculturation continuum: each older patient identified as a member of an "ethnic group" likely lives in a multicultural society, at some point between the extremes of being completely "traditional" based on her original culture, and completely "acculturated" to the American way of life; her position on the acculturation continuum will vary based on changing circumstances or social settings.
   - Intraethnic variation: the older patient lives a life experience that is unique and only approximates some notion of the imagined, complete ethnic culture.
7. Culture is sometimes *implicit.* Culture can be so embedded that the person cannot recognize some very important cultural dynamics and may even deny their existence.
8. The concept of *intercultural dynamics* operationalizes the realities of multicultural geriatric practice and avoids the subtle but real dynamic implicit in many attempts at cultural sensitivity, namely that "they" possess certain cultural oddities for which "we" must make adjustments in order to get compliance. This is an extremely biased approach and, while seeming to have the hallmarks of cultural sensitivity, it paradoxically serves to impede real intercultural communication.

Epidemiology of Geriatric Diseases by Ethnic and Racial Differences. It should be acknowledged that differences in health risks found in comparing ethnic populations in the U.S. are much less evident when studies control for differences in socioeconomic status. Nevertheless, knowledge of differential healthrisks, whatever their source, is important for providers to adequately screen older patients and learn to diagnose and manage the common conditions in a culturally competent manner. Table 8.2 illustrates

Table 8.2 Probable Differences in Health Risks Among Ethnic Elders Compared to Total Older U.S. Population, 1990[35–38] (– = lower than average; + = higher than average)

Type of Risk	Am. Indian/ Alaskan Nat.	Asian/Pacific Islander	Black	Hispanic
Cancer				
Combined	+		ma. +	Mex. –
Lung				Mex.ma. –
Breast				Mex.fe. +
Liver		Chin. +		Mex.fe. – PR +
Esophageal	+	Chin. + Jpn.ma. +		
Gallbladder	+			
Pancreatic		Chin.fe +		Mex.fe. +
Stomach		Jpn. +		Mex. +
Cervical			fe. +	Mex.fe. +
Prostate			ma. +	
Cardiac & Cardio-vascular Disease				
Heart Disease		Jpn.ma. +	fe. +	PR fe. +
Myocardial Infarction			ma. +	
Hypertension		Jpn.fe. – Fil. +	+	
CHF		Pac.Is. +	+	
Stroke			+	
Cataracts	+			
Dementia				
Alzheimer's			–	
Multi-Infarct		Chin. + Jpn. +	+	
Parkinson's		Guam. +		
Diabetes	+	Jpn. + Fil. + Pac.Is. +	+	Mex. + PR +
Depression		SE As. +		fem. +
Glaucoma			ma. +	
Gout		Fil. +		
Hearing problems	+			
Kidney Disease	+			
Liver Disease	+			
Obesity		Pac.Is. +	fe. +	Mex. +
Osteoporosis		Jpn. +		
(Hip Fracture)			fe. –	fe. –
Suicide		Chin.fe + Jpn. +	–	
Tuberculosis	+			
Undernutrition	Nav.ma. +			
Unintentional Injury	+			
Vision problems	+			

Legend: ma.=males; fe.=females; Chin.=Chinese; Fil.=Filipino; Guam.=Guamanian; Jpn.=Japanese; Mex.=Mexican; Nav.=Navaho; Pac.Is.=Pacific Islander; PR=Puerto Rican; SE As.=Southeast Asian.

risks for classes of conditions for elders from ethnic minority categories. Only conditions which have been found in at least one study to be significantly different for elders in the ethnic categories compared to the total or white population of U. S. elders are included.[35, 36, 37, 38]

Culturally Appropriate Geriatric Health Care. Although a comprehensive *fund of knowledge* is desirable for cultural competence in geriatric care, at a minimum, providers should understand: 1) major systems of culturally based health beliefs and values; and 2) historical experiences of the older cohorts of the larger ethnic populations.[39, 40]

While accurate geriatric *assessment* depends heavily on good communication and a thorough history, these may be difficult at best with elders who have immigrated from other countries, especially if the provider does not speak the language of a monolingual elder. Although family members are often used as *translators*, they should be used only as a last resort if a trained translator or translation service is not available, and then with caution. In cross gender discussion of topics that are taboo, such as the breast or genito-urinary organs a family member may change an inappropriate question or not ask it, so that the response is not accurate. When younger family members are asked to translate, it can be especially traumatic; they frequently feel inadequate or awkward if questions are seen to be demeaning to an elder or they are asked to give grave news. Even if a non-family translator is used, fear of being shamed or stigmatized if health information were leaked to the community may compromise responses on sensitive topics such as sex or mental illness. Use of translators is a skill frequently missing but vitally important in ethnogeriatric education.

Standardized assessment instruments are frequently used in geriatric practice, especially for areas such as mental status and depression, and have traditionally presented major obstacles to accurate assessment in ethnic minority elders. There are serious concerns around the translations and adaptation of standard assessment instruments. Mere translations are not acceptable but must be demonstrated to be valid and reliable with a new population. According to Geisinger[41] essential steps to insure that a translated test continues to measure the same characteristics include: 1) translation and adaptation of the measures with attention to fluency in language and specific cultural knowledge; 2) review of the translated or adapted version of the instrument by expert panel in a face to face meeting; 3) revision of the draft instrument based upon this discussion; 4) pilot testing of the revised draft with the population of interest and appropriate revisions based on results such as literacy level and misunderstandings of questions; 5) field testing and examination of internal consistency, test-retest issues, and response biases; 6) standardization of scores on the group of interest; 7) validation research (if appropriate); 8) development of manuals and documentation; 9) user training; and 10) ongoing collection of data from users. Recently, there has been increasing interest in developing and validating culturally and linguistically appropriate translations or adaptations of geriatric assessments, and the their availability for the larger ethnic groups is increasing rapidly.

Two approaches are available for use by geriatric providers in *assessing the intercultural dynamics* in clinical work.

1. In the "Itemized Belief System Elicitation" providers use one of several short questionnaires to elicit relevant

cultural elements that can be helpful in managing symptoms or gaining compliance. Recommendation by Kleinman and colleagues[42] to elicit patients' culturally based explanatory models of illness include: (1) What do you think has caused your problem? (2) Why do you think it started when it did? (3) What do you think your sickness does to you? How does it work? (4) How severe is your sickness? Will it have a short or long course? (5) What kind of treatment do you think you should receive? Others questions that may be incorporated if needed are: (6) What are the most important results you hope to receive from this treatment? (7) What are the chief problems your sickness has caused for you? and (8) What do you fear most about your sickness? Similar sets of questions are suggested by other authors, including Tripp-Reimer and colleagues,[43] who review nine different cultural assessment guides in the nursing literature.

Strengths of this approach include its brevity and ease of use, but an elder's culture is too complex to be well elicited by such a truncated method. Other limitations are the lack of consideration of the provider's or health system culture and a lack of guidance in interpreting elicited information.

2. In the "Deduction of Cultural Factors and Ranking of Importance" approach, the provider listens for relevant information in the history which can be categorized according to a check list for "cultural identity" systems, such as age, gender, or religion. The provider ranks the importance of the cultural aspects and integrates the most relevant factors with biomedical considerations.[44] Although this method is a means of beginning to make sense of cultural factors inherent in an elder's discourse and to track change over time, there are no specific prompts provided and the successful identification of cultural aspects is related to a provider's skill.

Until recently it was assumed that no physiological differences influence the effectiveness of *treatment* of particular groups of ethnic minority elders, once an accurate diagnosis was established; there is increasing evidence, however, that there may be important differences in response to medications among racial groups. The work of the scholars at the National Institute of Mental Health Research Center on the Psychobiology of Ethnicity at the University of California, Los Angeles, has shown that some medications in common classes used in geriatric care, such as antidepressants, benzodiazepines, and neuroleptics may produce different effects among different ethnic groups.[45]

The need and method of integrating information on *alternative (non-Western) treatments* that might have a bearing on Western therapeutic interventions (e.g., taking herbal remedies with diuretic effects) is completely missing in the geriatric medicine and allied health curricula with the exception of a few pharmacy programs. As a consequence, little or no attention is given by the vast majority of providers to inquiring about non-Western health remedies older ethnic patients (or majority elders, for that matter) might be taking, and few elders volunteer the information.

It has long been recognized that effective care for frail geriatric patients most often involves *working with family members* to jointly manage common chronic conditions and provide support for Activities of Daily Living and Instrumental Activities of Daily Living. In order for that care to be culturally competent, providers need to recognize the cultural expectations of families regarding aging relatives that guide the family members' responses. Areas that have been found to be particularly problematic for some ethnic minority families in their interface with medical providers have been the difference between Western providers and some ethnic families on the emphasis on "independence" as a goal of therapy; whether or not the elder should be told that he or she has a serious or life-threatening illness; how to reconcile the strong cultural norm that parents should always be cared for at home with the reality of lack of available family caregivers; ethical decision making with regard to life sustaining treatments for elders when providers predict little or no hope for recovery and religious beliefs teach faith in God to control the time and circumstances of death and/or faith in miracles.[46] Families faced with treatment decisions are frequently influenced strongly by their trust in their health care provider, which is in turn strongly influenced not only by the past collective experience of the ethnic group with the health care system (e.g., discrimination or experimentation), but also the degree to which the family feels understood culturally and individually.

3. Cross-Cultural Geriatric Training in Community-Based Education

Elders from ethnic groups are more likely to live in community settings, including living alone with support provided by friends or family, with their family, on a reservation, or in senior housing. They are less likely to be in nursing homes or other institutions. It is critical for providers to develop partnerships with family caregivers to provide effective care for the elders and support for the caregivers by linking them with community resources. Ethnogeriatric training of providers must be developed in partnership with the community through a service-learning emphasis; students would provide needed services while learning cultural issues for specific groups.

4. Support of Faculty Development in Ethnogeriatrics

Since few geriatric faculty have special training in ethnic issues, it is critical that special emphasis be given to the development of academic and clinical faculty with expertise to mentor students and provide good role models. In some cases this would be facilitated by medical anthropologists as members of the faculty to provide consultation. The following funded programs would be very helpful to support faculty development in ethnogeriatrics: 1) special mini-fellowships or mini-residencies in ethnogeriatrics to provide the expertise for at least one faculty member in each health care training program in geriatrics to develop cultural competence so that the knowledge and skills can then be taught to other key faculty; 2) Centers of Excellence in Ethnogeriatrics to serve as national resource and teaching centers for faculty; 3) development of multimedia resources and other innovative technology for teaching ethnogeriatrics to support trained faculty.

5. Support of Research in Ethnogeriatric Education

The public mandate for government to fund programs that are effective, accountable, and cost-effective requires an examination of the quality, appropriateness and effectiveness of geriatric health care education. Evaluation research is crucial to assess the outcomes of the following characteristics of ethnogeriatric education: 1) the number of ethnic minorities who pursue geriatrics; 2) the competence of geriatric specialists who work with minority populations; 3) model training programs for care of high-risk ethnic minority elders; 4) interdisciplinary team training models using cultural specialists; 5) ethnogeriatric fellowship programs; and 6) mentoring programs for both ethnic minority trainees and ethnogeriatric specialists.

6. Support of an Infrastructure to Integrate Ethnogeriatric Education into the Ongoing System of Education in Multiple Disciplines

Limitations on the integration of ethnogeriatric issues into health educational systems have been most evident in curriculum development, research, and program development. Other less obvious but equally important constituencies that must address these concerns include: legislators; national, regional, and local agencies; accrediting and licensing bodies; professional associations; research and program funding agencies; and administration. To provide the most comprehensive and effective health care to ethnogeriatric populations, all players must approach this topic with a focused, coordinated approach to enhance the educational training of health professionals and educators for cultural competence. Especially important for the institutionalization of ethnogeriatric curriculum is attention from the state and national boards who have responsibility for accrediting training programs in the respective disciplines and for developing and implementing examinations to license and relicense health professionals. Not until ethnogeriatrics is included in these evaluations which legitimize the standards of health professions training will the need for cultural competence be taken seriously by students and faculty alike.

The goal of cultural competence training in geriatric care is to develop the ability to understand and integrate the distinct and various cultural values, beliefs, and behaviors into the proposed plan of action for health care. To this end, recommendations are directed toward policy makers at all levels who have direct input into the development of health care systems.

RECOMMENDATIONS

Recruitment, Training, and Retention

1. Increase the numbers of geriatric specialists such as physicians, nurses, social workers, occupational therapists, physical therapists, psychologists, and others, who are members of ethnic minority groups and able to provide ethnically competent practice.

Rationale

It is an unnecessary tragedy for this ever-graying nation to lose ethnic minority geriatric health care personnel resources due to social, cultural, political, or economic factors. Among many ethnic minority youth, the perception exists that health sciences training is an unattainable occupational wish. Such perceptions reduce the prospect of self-selection for health sciences training among ethnic minority youth at the same numbers proportionally found in the majority population. Among currently practicing professionals, there is a marked need to train ethnic minority professionals for geriatric competence. The presence of such professionals serves as role models and landmarks for attracting others who have experienced American life in a culturally specific way different than the mainstream. Yet, the presence of ethnic minority professionals who are geriatric specialists does not automatically confer ethnogeriatric competence. Consequently, there remains a strong need to further educate geriatric specialists in competent care for ethnic minority patients.

Action Required

1) Recruitment and retention of ethnic minority students into the health professions with a geriatric focus must be intensified by including geriatrics in programs which have ethnic minority recruitment for health professions. This targets junior high and high schools as well as undergraduate colleges. For example, within these educational institutions, offices for Health Careers Opportunity programs and Minority Action Research Centers should be focal points for recruitment and retention.
2) Ethnic minority professionals currently practicing in geriatrics must be identified and recruited into continuing education courses which will teach ethnic competence practice skills.
3) Fellowships with stipend support, tuition payment/waivers, and payback agreements must be increased in order to significantly increase the numbers of ethnic minorities who pursue ethnogeriatrics as a career.

Responsible Agents

1) National associations of high school guidance counseling offices; Association of Gerontology in Higher Education; Health Resources and Services Administration; National Institutes of Health.
2) Nationally distributed Geriatric Education Centers; American Geriatric Society; Gerontological Society of America; American Society on Aging; university programs.
3) Congressional mandate to set aside money for education and training of ethnic minorities in geriatrics at the Fellowship level across all disciplines.

Expected Outcomes

1) Within 10 years, there will be an increase to their proportions in the populations in numbers of ethnic minorities who are recruited and retained to pursue health sciences careers with a geriatric focus;
2) Within 3 years, there will be an increase in those receiving ethnogeriatric training at Geriatric Education Centers, professional geriatric and gerontological organizations, and university programs, and
3) receive financial assistance pursuant to geriatric and ethnogeriatric health care training and service.

2. Develop Centers of Excellence in Ethnogeriatrics which conduct special intensive training in geriatrics.

Rationale

By providing the expertise for at least one faculty member in each health care training program in geriatrics to develop cultural competence, their knowledge and skills can then be taught to other key faculty. Training in ethnogeriatrics resulting in real cultural competence requires an intensive educational experience lead by experts in the field. A critical mass of such expertise needs to be organized into a coordinated network of Centers of Excellence in Ethnogeriatrics. Moreover, valuable time can be saved using a "train-the-trainer" approach when applied in an intensive training program.

Action Required

In order to conduct intensive training in ethnogeriatrics to meet the abundant and expanding national need, educational resource centers need to be developed as "Centers of Excellence in Ethnogeriatrics." At least six such centers will be developed and distributed regionally.

Responsible Agents

Congress, the Bureau of Health Professions

in partnership with foundations (e.g., Robert Wood Johnson, Kellogg, Pew, Commonwealth, and Andrus).

Expected Outcomes

Within 3 years, Congress will allocate funds to establish a network of at least six regionally distributed Centers of Excellence in Ethnogeriatrics. Within 2 years of start-up of the Centers, newly trained graduates will begin teaching ethnogeriatric skills to their faculty and students.

Ethnogeriatric Curriculum

3. A curriculum in ethnogeriatrics must be required as part of the core knowledge and skills practice base of all health professions caring for older adults.

Rationale

In order to improve the services, service utilization, and quality of care received by all elders in terms of their cultural backgrounds, a core ethnogeriatric curriculum is required in geriatrics training. Infusion of such a core ethnogeriatric curriculum in geriatrics will reach health science students early in their training. As a core part of curriculum, ethnogeriatrics will be viewed as essential content from early in the training.

Action Required

1) Health care professional licensing and accreditation organizations will include ethnogeriatrics in their requirements;
2) Develop and implement a core ethnogeriatric curriculum supported by licensure and accreditation organizations for all the health professions disciplines that incorporates at the minimum the following areas (see above section on Vision for details):

- Learning objectives and theoretical base
- Content
    - Intercultural dynamics
    - Epidemiology of geriatric diseases by race/ethnic group
    - Culturally appropriate geriatric health care
      ***Background Information*:** a) major systems of culturally based health beliefs; b) historical experiences of the older cohorts of the major populations
      ***Skills*:** a) use of translators; b) assessment instruments; c) assessment of intercultural dynamics; d) treatment/management issues including differences in responses to medications, coordination with non-Western therapies, and working with families from diverse cultures; and *Ethical Decision Making*.
- Instructional strategies
- Evaluation methods

Responsible Agents

1) Professional accreditation organizations and curriculum committees in the health sciences schools;
2) the regional Centers of Excellence in Ethnogeriatrics; curriculum develop will be assisted by the National Association of Geriatric Education Centers in partnership with relevant professional organizations; funding will be made available by foundations and the Bureau of Health Professions; Educational networks within health professions organizations;

Expected Outcomes

Within 3 years, a minimum of three health care professions licensing and accreditation organizations will include ethnogeriatrics in their requirements;
2) Within 3 years, revision of curriculum

and its implementation, will be implemented in a minimum of three health professions.

4. Community-based providers and institutionally based educators must become partners on curriculum committees and as community preceptors responsible for the integration of ethnogeriatric curricula into larger curricula.

Rationale

Professionals working in ethnic minority communities are valuable resources as role models for trainees. Partnership between the educational institution and practitioners participating in an ethnic minority community yields a powerful product of principle and realism. Such interactions constitute a valuable experience with which to enrich the basic principles of ethnic minority elder geriatric curriculum development. Professionals working in ethnic minority communities can offer realistic, practice-based expertise to trainees. Building collaborative relationships with existing community agencies who have been providing health and social services to ethnic minority elders will enhance and strengthen the trainees' experience.

Action Required

1) Develop and disseminate guidelines for involving appropriate community based providers;
2) identify appropriate community based providers for recruitment onto curriculum committees.

Responsible Agents

1) Geriatric Education Centers;
2) aging services network; professional accreditation organizations; faculty with knowledge of the community-based health care environment can identify candidates for curriculum committee involvement.

Expected Outcomes

1) Within 5 years, there will be an increased number of community based providers involved in curriculum development;
2) Within 5 years, universities will be utilizing an increased number of community based providers to serve as preceptors for training.

5. Development and marketing of multimedia resources and other innovative technology for teaching ethnogeriatrics should be developed to support trained faculty.

Rationale

In order for ethnogeriatrics to be sustained as core content in the health sciences curriculum, there must be curricular support. Such support includes resources in terms of curriculum guides, media of all types, and widely available, well marketed information on where to get additional and ongoing curricular assistance. Presently, resources are limited and mostly unavailable. Ethnogeriatric curriculum information can be easily collected, maintained, and disseminated from central facilities such as data banks. There will be ongoing improvements in the means by which to teach the substantive content as well as methods to use.

Action Required

Development of materials in support of ongoing ethnogeriatric education.

Responsible Agents

Centers of Excellence in Ethnogeriatrics, Geriatric Education Centers, commercial enterprises such as publishing companies, and Small Business Innovation Research projects of National Institute of Aging and the National Institute of Mental Health related to ethnogeriatric development.

Expected Outcome

Within 5 years, ethnogeriatric material will be made available for use in curriculum development by Centers of Excellence in Ethnogeriatrics, Geriatric Education Centers, commercial companies, and the Small Business Innovation Research projects of National Institute of Aging and the National Institute of Mental Health related to ethnogeriatric development.

6. The structure for ongoing support of ethnogeriatrics as a fundamental part of the core health sciences curricula must be put in place, including accrediting of training programs and licensing of health professions.

Rationale

The value of ethnogeriatrics in an aging, multicultural society is enormous. Yet, change from the current standard to an improved one can be difficult. Therefore, the implementation of comprehensive change in existing educational systems such as universities and curriculum related licensing and accreditation organizations must be accomplished at foundational levels so that, in this case, new ethnogeriatric capabilities will become integrated and routinized. Without real support at the roots of the geriatric educational system, there is a strong risk that only a thin veneer of ethnogeriatric training improvement will occur. The inclusion of ethnogeriatric concepts at the decision making level of educational development in the health sciences will assist in the integration of ethnogeriatrics as part of the expected and required fabric of geriatric health science education.

Action Required

Members of licensing and accreditations organizations and university education committees must become cognizant of the importance and demand for ethnogeriatric knowledge and skills.

Responsible Agents

Licensing and accreditation organizations; educational committees of professional associations; Bureau of Health Professions and the Pew Foundation.

Expected Outcomes

Within five years, ethnogeriatrics will be a requisite aspect of accreditation and licensing organizations and university educational committees.

Evaluation Research

7. Standardized evaluation should become a component in all funded training and educational programs relative to ethnogeriatrics.

Rationale

In order to address public and Congressional concerns about the accountability, efficacy, and cost-effectiveness of specific educational issues, appropriate data must be collected on ethnogeriatric curricular programs. Inclusion of standard evaluation components will significantly enhance research in search of excellence in ethnogeriatrics training because national data can be pooled. Critical evaluation data can help training programs, federal agencies and the public insure that effective programs are supported. Also, research on ethnogeriatric training issues will guide the continuous improvement of ethnogeriatric curricular development.

Action Required

Federal agencies develop standard education and training evaluation tools and mandate collection in funding requirements. Develop national data base of evaluation data. Results of evaluation research will be made available to others.

Responsible Agents

Bureau of Health Professions as well as other federal agencies, and the Centers for Excellence in Ethnogeriatrics.

Expected Outcomes

Within 2 years of implementation, measurable improvement in training and educational programs in ethnogeriatrics will be available.

8. Interdisciplinary team models in ethnogeriatrics and mentorship programs for ethnic minority trainees should be developed, implemented, and evaluated.

Rationale

There is a public mandate for government to fund programs that are effective, accountable, and cost-effective. This mandate translates into an examination into the quality, appropriateness and effectiveness of health care services through a broad program of scientific research and information dissemination. Interdisciplinary team models and mentorship programs are identified by experts as best-practice models in ethnogeriatric education. However, little empirical research is available to support this assumption.

Action Required

1) Collect information about interdisciplinary and mentorship programs which includes curriculum guidelines and resources; 2) develop, fund, and evaluate educational and curriculum replication projects in ethnogeriatrics around the country. This funding can be directed toward the Centers of Excellence in Ethnogeriatrics.

Responsible Agents

Bureau of Health Professions, Administration on Aging and other federal agencies that provide training support and foundations.

Expected Outcomes

1) Within 5 years there will be a minimum of six interdisciplinary and mentorship programs developed, implemented, and evaluated.
2) Within 10 years, there will be replication projects completed.

REFERENCES

1. U.S. Bureau of the Census & National Institute on Aging. Racial and ethnic diversity of America's elderly population. Profiles of America's Elderly. Washington, DC: Author, 1993
2. U.S. Census of Population and Housing. Summary of Tape File 1, California. Sacramento, CA: State of California State Census Data Center, 1990
3. California Department of Finance. Projected Total Population for California by Race/ Ethnicity. Sacramento, CA: Population Research Unit, 1988
4. Liu, WT & Yu E. Asian/Pacific American elderly: mortality differentials, health status and use of health services. J Applied Geront 1985; 4:35-64
5. Kastenbaum R. "Oh where, oh where has ethnicity gone?" In Gelfand, DE & Kutzik, AJ (Eds.) Ethnicity and Aging: Theory, Research, and Policy. New York: Springer, 1979
6. Yeo G. Ethnogeriatric education: need and content. J Cross-Cultural Geront 1991; 6:229–241
7. Peterson, DA, Bergstone D, & Lobenstine J. National Director of Educational Programs in Gerontology. Washington, DC: Association of Gerontology in Higher Education, 1987

8. Federal Register, Considerations for Grants for GECS. October, 1986
9. Federal Register. Considerations for Grants for GECS. October 7, 1988
10. Federal Register. Considerations for Grants for GECS. April 16, 1993
11. Harper, MS (Ed.) Minority Aging: Essential Curricula Content for Selected Health and Allied Health Professions. Health Resources and Services Administration, Department of Health and Human Services. DHHS Publication No. HRS (P-DV-90-4). Washington DC: U.S. Government Printing Office, 1990
12. Yeo G. Ethnogeriatric Curriculum and Training in Geriatric Education Centers. Geront Geriat Ed 1992; 12:40–48
13. Francis, D, Shenk D, & Sokolovsky J. Teaching About Aging: Interdisciplinary and Cross-Cultural Perspectives. Association for Anthropology and Gertontology, 1990
14. Gerontological Society of America. Minority Elders: Longevity, Economics, and Health. Washington, DC: Author, 1991
15. Gerontological Society of America (1994). Minority Elders: Five Goals Toward Building a Public Policy Base. Washington, DC: Author.
16. Bureau of Health Professions. GEC Materials Related to Minority Aging. Washington, DC: Author, 1994
17. Western Institute of Nursing (1991) Author.
18. McCormack, G, Llorens L, & Glogoski C. Culturally diverse elders. In Kiernat, J.M. (Ed.) Occupational therapy and the older adult. Gaithersburg, MD: Aspen, 1991
19. DeSylvia-Valenti, DA, Good GW, & Mancil GL. Managing low income and minority elderly patients. In Optometric Gerontology: A Resource Manual for Educators. Rockville, MD: Association of Schools and College of Optometry, 1992
20. Giordano J. Ethnicity and aging. In Mellor, J, & Solomon, R (Eds.) Geriatric Social Work Education. Binghamton, NY: Haworth Press (also Journal of Gerontological Social Work 18), 1992
21. Douglas, K. & Lenahan P. Ethnogeriatric assessment clinic in family medicine. Family Medicine 1994; 26:372–5
22. Wallace, S. The contribution of public health to gerontology: an evaluation of public health curricula on aging. Geront & Geriatr Ed 1994; 14:21–37
23. Wallace, S. & Prohaska TR. Introductory course developed at the 1992 public health and aging curriculum development workshop. In Proceedings from the Aging and Public Health Curriculum Development Workshop. Los Angeles: California GEC, 1993
24. Kleinman, A. Patients and Healers in the Context of Culture: An Exploration of the Borderland between Anthropology, Medicine, and Psychiatry. Berkeley: University of California Press, 1980
25. Leininger, M. Transcultural Nursing: Concepts, Theories, and Practice. New York: John Wiley & Sons, 1978
26. Yee, BWK. Variations in Aging: Older Minorities. Texas Consortium of Geriatric Education Centers, UTMB School of Allied Health Sciences, University of Texas Medical Branch at Galveston, U.S. DHHS Grant #5-D31AH66005-05 Bureau of Health Professions, Geriatrics/Gerontology Curriculum Module. 1st Ed, 1989, 2nd, 2990, 3rd Ed, 1991, 4th Ed, 1995
27. Lewin, ME & Rice B. (Eds.) Balancing the Scales of Opportunity: Ensuring Racial and Ethnic Diversity in the Health Professions. Committee on increasing Minority participation in the Health professions, Institute of Medicine, Washington D.C: National Academy Press. 1994
28. Scott-Jones. American Psychological Association (APA) Fellowship Program: Financial support and professional development. Paper presented in symposium "Minority Initiatives in APA: Have they worked?" Annual Meeting of the APA Washington D.C., August, 1992.
29. Jones, JM. Who is training our ethnic minority psychologists, and are they doing it right? In Stricker, G, Davis-Russell E,

Duran E, Hammond WR, McHolland J, Polite K, & Baughn BE (Eds.), Toward ethnic diversity in psychology education and training. Washington D.C.: American Psychological Association, 1990
30. Fowkes, V, Gamel N, Garcia R, & Wilson N. Assessment of Physician Assistant, Nurse Practitioner, and Nurse Midwife Training on Meeting Health Care Needs of the Underserved. Final Report to Bureau of Health Professions. Palo Alto CA: Division of Family and Community Medicine, Stanford University, 1993
31. Levkoff, S & Berkman B. Strategies of minority recruitment among Geriatric Education Centers. Geront Geriatr Ed 1992; 12:29–40.
32. Berlin, EA and Fowkes WC. A teaching framework for cross-cultural health care. Western J Med 1983; 139:934–938
33. Henderson, N. The "cultural diversity" epidemic. Editiorial. Gerontological Health Section Newsletter. American Public Health Association, 1993
34. Borkan, JM. & Nehar JO. A developmental model of ethnosensitivity in family practice training. Family Med 1991; 23:212–217
35. McCabe, M & Cuellar J. Aging and Health: American Indian/Alaska Native Elders, 2nd. SGEC Working Paper #6. Stanford, CA: Stanford GEC, 1994
36. Morioka-Douglas, N. & Yeo G. Aging and Health: Asian/Pacific Island American Elders SGEC Working Paper #3. Stanford, CA: Stanford GEC, 1990
37. Richardson, J. Aging and Health: Black American Elders. SGEC Working Paper #4. Stanford, CA:Stanford GEC, 1990
38. Villa, ML, Cuellar J, Gamel N, & Yeo G. Aging and Health: Hispanic American Elders, 2nd. SGEC Working Paper #5. Stanford, CA: SGEC
39. G. Ethnogeriatric education: need and recommendations. In Shortage of Health Care Professions Caring for the Elderly: Recommendations for Change. A Report by the Chairman of the Select Committee on Aging House of Representatives. Washington, DC: U.S. Govt. Printing Office, 1992.
40. Baker, FM & Lightfoot O. Psychiatric care of ethnic elders. In Gaw, AC (Ed.) Culture, Ethnicity, and Mental Illness. Washington, DC: American Psychiatric Press, 1993
41. Geisinger, KF. Cross-cultural normative assessment: Translation and adaptation issues influencing the normative interpretation of assessment instruments. Psychological Assessment 1994;6: 304–312
42. Kleinman, A,. Eisenberg L, & Good B. Culture, illness, and care: clinical lessons from anthropologic and cross-cultural research. Ann Internal Med 1978; 88:251
43. Tripp-Reimer, T, Brink PJ, & Saunders JM Cultural assessment: content and process. Nursing Outlook 1984; 32:78–82
44. Hill, R. F., J. D. Fortenberyy, and H. F. Stein. Culture in clinical medicine. Southern Medical J 1991; 83:1071–1080
45. Lin, K-M, Poland R & Nakasaki G. Psychopharmacology and Psychobiology of Ethnicity. New York: American Psychiatry Press, 1993
46. Kim, S. Ethnic elders and American health care—a physician's perspective. J Western Med 1983; 139:885–891